The Health of China

The Health of China

Ruth Sidel and Victor W. Sidel

with a chapter on education by Mark Sidel

Beacon Press ● Boston

Portions of this book were drawn from Ruth Sidel, *Women and Child Care in China: A Firsthand Report* (Baltimore: Penguin, 1973); Victor W. Sidel and Ruth Sidel, *Serve the People: Observations on Medicine in the People's Republic of China* (Boston: Beacon Press, 1973); Ruth Sidel, *Families of Fengsheng: Urban Life in China* (Baltimore: Penguin Books, 1974); Victor W. Sidel and Ruth Sidel, *A Healthy State: An International Perspective on the Crisis in U.S. Medical Care* (New York: Pantheon, 1978); material that we prepared for the chapter on "Health and Human Services" and Mark Sidel prepared for "The Educational System" in *Encyclopedia for China Today* by Fredric M. Kaplan and Julian Sobin (New York: Eurasia Press, 1981).

Beacon Press books are published under the auspices
of the Unitarian Universalist Association, 25 Beacon
Street, Boston, Massachusetts 02108

Published simultaneously in Canada by
Fitzhenry & Whiteside Limited, Toronto

Printed in the United States of America

(hardcover) 9 8 7 6 5 4 3 2 1

Library of Congress Cataloging in Publication Data

Sidel, Ruth, 1933–
    The health of China

    Bibliography: p.
    Includes index.
    1. Public health–China. 2. Public welfare–
China. 3. Medical policy–China. 4. China–
Social policy. I. Sidel, Victor W., 1931-
II. Sidel, Mark. III. Title.
RA527.S495   362.1′0951   81-68353
ISBN 0-8070-2160-1   AACR2

To Edgar
a brother and a friend
with our love

A European lately arrived in China, if he is of a receptive and reflective disposition, finds himself confronted with a number of very puzzling questions, for many of which the problems of Western Europe will not have prepared him . . . Chinese problems, even if they affected no one outside China, would be of vast importance, since the Chinese are estimated to constitute about a quarter of the human race. In fact, however, all the world will be vitally affected by the development of Chinese affairs, which may well prove a decisive factor, for good or evil, during the next two centuries. This makes it important, to Europe and America almost as much as to Asia, that there should be an intelligent understanding of the questions raised by China, even if, as yet, definite answers are difficult to give.

> Bertrand Russell
> *The Problem of China,* 1922

From my studies of the development problems in underdeveloped countries I have reached the conclusion that there is no conflict between the goals of growth and social justice. Instead, radical egalitarian reforms are a necessary condition for sustained growth and development.

> Gunnar Myrdal
> "Growth and Social Justice"
> *World Development,* 1973

Acknowledgments

We are grateful to the Chinese Medical Association for its hospitality during our four visits to China. It was through the painstaking efforts of the staff of the Association that we have been able to visit and, even more important, repeatedly revisit communes, neighborhoods, medical facilities, schools, and factories over the past decade. Two people in China have been of extraordinary help to us in our efforts to understand the Chinese experience: Professor Yang Mingding, Head, Faculty of Public Health, Shanghai First Medical College, and Dr. Xu Jiayu, Deputy Chairman, Department of Internal Medicine, Ruijin Hospital, Shanghai Second Medical College. We are grateful to them for their wisdom and their friendship. We are also deeply grateful to the following for facilitating our work in China: Gu Dezhang, Chinese Medical Association, Peking; Dr. Liu Xiangyun, Director, Shanghai Children's Hospital; Dr. Wang Hongzhen, Deputy Director, Shanghai Public Health Bureau; and Zhang Shuyi, Secretary-General, Chinese People's National Committee for the Defense of Children, Peking.

We are indebted to James Peck for his illuminating discussions with us about developments in China and for reviewing part of the manuscript; to Dr. Shu Yijing, Dr. Molly Coye, and Daniel Lindheim for comments on specific chapters; to Dr. Roberto Belmar for helping us to clarify issues of primary health care around the world and for his ever-present revolutionary optimism; and to Kevin Sidel for his continuing stimulation and support. At Beacon Press, we thank MaryAnn Lash, who was extremely helpful in planning this book, and Jeff Smith and Judy Rosen, who have helped bring it to fruition. Among those who worked on repeated drafts of the manuscript, we thank Barbara Aiken, Helen O'Brien, Eve Teitelbaum, Edythe Weber, and Phoebe Weber.

Mark Sidel not only contributed a chapter to this book but also, using his fluency in the Chinese language and his knowledge gained from living in China, commented on much of the manuscript. Any errors in this book are ours; any useful insights must be credited, at least in part, to his depth of understanding of current events in China.

Introduction

China's work in health and human services burst upon the United States and indeed the world in 1971. After a period of sixteen years, starting in 1949, during which little attention was paid to China's progress, followed by six years during which visitors from other countries were rare—and visitors from the United States essentially non-existent—China's invitation to a United States Ping-Pong team playing in an international tournament in Japan signaled a new era in China's relations with other countries. Within a few months Henry Kissinger had visited Peking to prepare the way for President Nixon's 1972 visit. The breakthrough occurred largely because both Washington and Peking viewed their foreign policy interests as better served by a lessening of the hostility of the previous twenty years and by the beginning of a rapprochement between the two nations. In the current jargon, the U.S. played its "China card" and China played its U.S. card; the nation against which both were playing was, of course, the Soviet Union.

The breakthrough in what had been called the "bamboo curtain" was followed by a trickle and then a stream of visitors from the United States and other countries. Visits by citizens of China to other countries began much more slowly, but increased during the decade. In the wake of the exchange of visitors there was an enormous flood of interest in what had been happening, what was happening, and what was going to happen in China. The fact that this interest was perceived as serving U.S. foreign policy—in diminishing the vast gulf of mistrust that had developed—encouraged the media in the U.S. to provide heavy coverage of events in China. The media of other countries joined in the general stampede to publish, broadcast, photograph, and ultimately sell all things Chinese.

Reliable information from Western observers—including material on health care—had of course been available prior to 1971. Edgar Snow's visits to China had continued and his accounts of his travels and observations throughout China and his discussions with Chinese leaders were widely read.[1] In medicine, Joshua Horn, a British orthopedic surgeon, had published accounts of his unique fifteen-year experience of living and practicing medicine in China.[2] And other visitors—such as Canadian doctors, invited because of the special relationship between China and Canada engendered by the work of the Canadian thoracic surgeon Norman Bethune in the late 1930s and by continuing diplomatic relations and trade between the two countries—had published accounts of medical care in China.[3] But it wasn't until the early 1970s that the media of the U.S. and its allies, taking their cue from the U.S. State Department, spread China's accomplishments before a waiting world.

The success of this effort to change public opinion about China was astounding. In a Gallup Poll in 1966, a representative sample of the American people were asked to choose adjectives that best describe the people of specific other countries. The adjectives most frequently selected for the Chinese people were "hardworking," "warlike," "ignorant," "sly," and "treacherous." In a similar poll in 1972, the adjectives most frequently chosen to describe the Chinese people were "hardworking," "intelligent," "progressive," "practical," and "artistic."[4]

It is not surprising that advances in health and other human services were specifically chosen by the Chinese to illustrate dramatically the progress China had made since the Communists took power in 1949. In September 1971, five months after the visit of the Ping-Pong team, the Chinese Medical Association—technically a nongovernmental body but in actuality closely intertwined with the Chinese Ministry of Public Health—invited the first U.S. medical delegation in twenty years to visit China. We were fortunate to be part of that small group. The Chinese Medical Association was our host because, in the absence of diplomatic relations between the U.S. and China, the visit was considered by the Chinese as "people to people" rather than governmental.

On our return from visits to Peking, Shanghai, Guangzhou (Canton), and Hangzhou (Hangchow), including a meeting that Premier Zhou Enlai (Chou En-lai) held with all the Americans who were in China at that time, we were greeted from the moment we crossed the border into Hong Kong with extraordinary demands for information and analysis on what we had seen in China. This visit was followed by invitations to return to China in 1972 (with our two sons), in 1977, and our most recent visit in the summer of 1980.

Reports of the incredible progress the Chinese had made in health care, their care of children, particularly preschool children, and the provision of human services within intricately organized urban neighborhoods astonished and gave hope to Americans of all ages and political persuasions who had begun to despair about finding humane solutions to human problems in our postindustrial society. Reports out of China about the Chinese policy of "self-reliance" and "walking on two legs" also gave hope to people in other nations, particularly in the third world, to whom it had become clear that "trickle-down" development policies were not solving the problems of extreme poverty and maldistribution of resources but were enriching the "haves" at the expense of the "have-nots." Here, suddenly, was another model of modernization, one that had clear relevance to poor, largely rural third world nations.

The World Bank—in its *World Development Report 1981*—summarized the international view of China's progress:

> . . . China's most remarkable achievement during the past three decades has been to make low-income groups far better off in terms of basic needs than their counterparts in most other poor countries. They all have work; their food supply is guaranteed through a mixture of state rationing and collective self-insurance; most of their children are not only at school but are also being comparatively well taught; and the great majority have access to basic health care and family planning services. Life expectancy— whose dependence on many other economic and social variables makes it probably the best single indicator of the extent of real poverty in a country—is (at 64 years) outstandingly high for a country at China's per capita income level . . .[5]

Many international agencies quickly adopted aspects of the Chinese developmental model for use in their work. The World Health Organization (WHO), for example, had, for the most part, since its inception in 1948 been sending consultants on "high-quality" technological services to poor countries and supporting the building of urban "centers of excellence" from which, it was assumed, well-trained people and good technology would diffuse into the rural areas and into poor urban areas. That this model was failing to accomplish its purpose was evident before 1971, but implications of the alternative Chinese model encouraged a rapid reversal. WHO published—and advocated—a variety of materials and models either directly based on or closely related to China's approaches to health services. Examples included changes in language and style (from "technical assistance" to "technical cooperation"); publication of books like *Health By the People* and other materials on decentralized health services using indigenous health workers similar to China's barefoot doctors; advocacy through multiple media of the integration of traditional medicine with modern medicine; and the adoption of new priorities such as "primary health care" and "health for all by the year 2000."[6] Articles began to appear specifically discussing the applicability of Chinese models to other developing countries. One example, in the widely read British medical journal *The Lancet,* was entitled "Is the Chinese 'Barefoot Doctor' Exportable to Rural Iran?" The answer was "no," unless other structural changes in Iran were accomplished, but the attempt to use the Chinese model had been made.[7] It is now difficult to find an analysis of health care in the third world that does not refer, explicitly or implicitly, to China's experience.

Even in technologically developed countries there were many efforts to "learn from China." A number of aspects of health and other human services in affluent societies are clearly failing to meet people's needs in effective, efficient, and humane ways, and China appeared to offer both new ideas and inspiration for change. In the Bronx, for example, a program was initiated to train people living in local apartment buildings to work with their neighbors on health problems and disease prevention. The models for training and work of these "health coordinators" owed much to the patterns of training and work of the "Red Medical Workers" in China's cities.

Similarly, in the field of preschool care, teachers were moved upon learning of the Chinese efforts to promote cooperation and mutual caring among young children to attempt to develop similar techniques in their own society. Their work was consistently frustrated by the contradictions between their goals and the competitive, often uncaring, sometimes violent environment the children lived in, but reports of the Chinese experience had clarified their objectives and had made them seem attainable.

As the decade ended, however, it was seen as ironic that just as people in many of the world's countries began to explore the possibility of introducing radical new ideas from China into their own development plans and health and human services, China has appeared to pull back abruptly from the models it had been developing. There was great confusion among those who had attempted to learn from the Chinese experience: Was decentralization of services and extensive use of indigenous health and human service workers a good idea or was it not? Was integration of traditional medicine with modern medicine useful or not? Was emphasis on accessibility of health care to rural people and deemphasis on high-technology medicine the appropriate path for poor countries or was it simply a way of maintaining their backwardness? Would China's models of preschool care survive a rigid drive for "modernization"? Were the radical changes in education during the Cultural Revolution functional or were they simply an unsuccessful, transient experiment?

Unfortunately much of the material that appeared in the Chinese press—excoriation of the Gang of Four, description of the Cultural Revolution as "ten lost years," debate whether the policies of that period were "ultra-right," "ultra-left," or something else—was of little help to those in other countries who knew that their own national policies were largely counterproductive and led to an increasing rather than a diminishing gulf between the poor and the rich. Furthermore, China's proclivity for describing its changing policies either completely positively or completely negatively adds to the confusion in other countries' efforts to understand and evaluate China's experience. In short, as China's development policy abruptly changed, the rest of the world was left with the problem of trying to sort out what China's shift in policy meant for China's future and for policy formation in other countries.

In our 1977 and 1980 visits we therefore concentrated on observation of the changes that had occurred since our visits earlier in
the decade. We have been extremely fortunate—and almost unique—
in our opportunity to view with outsiders' perspectives the changes
in health and human services in China over an extraordinary ten years.
Since these services are so intricately intertwined with Chinese political
and economic ideology and practice, changes in these areas provide a
window on the broader developments within Chinese society. Those
changes and, insofar as we can fathom them, their origins and their
implications for the future are the topic of this book.

Technical Note

An explanatory note on transliteration and translation of Chinese characters may be useful. The transliteration used in this book follows whenever possible the *pinyin* system of Romanization, the system officially adopted for use in China. Exceptions are made where the use of *pinyin* would, in our opinion, obscure rather than clarify, as in the long-accepted use in the West of "Peking" rather than "Beijing" and "Kuomintang" rather than "Guomindang." Where there are other forms in common use but the *pinyin* now seems preferable, the familiar form is given in parentheses the first time the *pinyin* form is used, as in "Xian" ("Sian") and "Zhou Enlai" ("Chou En-lai"). As to translation of Chinese words, an attempt is made to use the common English expression or the official Chinese translation, but where meaning or nuance may be lost (as in the official translation of *zili gengsheng* as "self-reliance"), the alternative or literal meaning ("regeneration through one's own efforts") is given the first time the words are used. As another example, *xueyuan* is usually translated as "institute"; when it is used in the title of what is known in the United States as a medical "school," we translate it as "college." The word "school" cannot be used for this translation because it must be reserved for translation of the name of the "middle-level" institutions for the training of nurses, assistant doctors, and other health workers. Because transliteration and translation of Chinese terms within and outside China are often inconsistent and may cause confusion, non–Chinese-speaking visitors to China who are concerned about the precise meaning of a word should insist that the interpreter provide them with the Chinese character or its *pinyin* equivalent.

The letters used in *pinyin* are pronounced, in general, as they are in English; the major exceptions are:

c is pronounced as the ts in its

q is pronounced as the ch in cheek

x is pronounced as the sh in she

zh is pronounced as the j in jump[8]

Chinese currency (*Renminbi*) has as its basic unit the yuan (Y); a yuan is divided into 10 jiao and into 100 fen ("cents"). The exchange rate for the yuan in 1981 was U.S. $0.67; in other words, one U.S. dollar bought Y1.50.

Contents

Introduction xi

Technical Note xvii

I. From Mao to Modernization 1

 Chapter 1 — The Political Pendulum, 1971–1981 3

II. Health Care Services 17

 Chapter 2 — Four Millennia of Medicine 19

 Chapter 3 — Shoes for the Barefoot Doctor? 35

 Chapter 4 — Put Prevention First! 71

III. Human Services 99

 Chapter 5 — The Individual, the Group, the Community:
  Problems of Daily Life 101

 Chapter 6 — The Family and Child Care: The First Collective 125

 Chapter 7 — Education: "Red" versus "Expert" (Mark Sidel) 150

IV. China's and the World's Future 175

 Chapter 8 — Which Model for Modernization? 177

 Appendix A — Professional Medical Workers in China,
  1978–1980 208

 Appendix B — Barefoot Doctor Vocational Evaluation
  Test, Peking Municipality 210

 Appendix C — Institutes and Hospitals of the Chinese Academy
  of Medical Sciences and the Chinese Academy
  of Traditional Medicine, 1981 213

 Appendix D — Medical Colleges in China, 1980 215

 Appendix E — Reported Cases of Selected Infectious
  Diseases in China, 1978–1980 219

 Appendix F — Key Universities in China, 1980 220

 Appendix G — Institutes of the Chinese Academy
  of Social Sciences, 1980 223

 Notes 224

 Bibliography 240

 Index 243

I | From Mao to Modernization

1 | The Political Pendulum, 1971–1981

The China that we visited in 1971 and 1972 was a society in the process of reorganizing its social institutions in the wake of the most turbulent years of the Cultural Revolution. The period from 1966 to 1969 was a time of massive political upheaval, of profound reexamination of methods and goals, and of a power struggle between the forces of Mao Zedong and the forces of Liu Shaoqi, the head of state of the People's Republic of China since 1959. It was a period during which, in the Chinese phrase, the entire country was exhorted to "put politics in command." It was a period of reevaluating the role of Communist party officials, of the bureaucracy, and of specialists in all fields. It was a period of attempting to shift resources from the urban areas to the far poorer countryside, of attempting to break down some of the traditional barriers between mental and physical labor and between intellectuals on the one hand and workers and peasants on the other. It was a time of glorification of those who prior to 1949 were the most oppressed: the workers, the peasants, and the soldiers. In sum, the increasing disparity between resources in the countryside and those in the city, the widening gulf between intellectuals and those who worked with their hands, and the separation between government and Party officials and the people were, we were told in 1971 and 1972, the central issues of the Cultural Revolution.

3

The chief instigator of the Cultural Revolution, it was emphasized in the 1970s, was Mao himself. The great revolutionary leader of the Chinese people, the architect of the 1949 Liberation and of the new Chinese state, he had put his unique influence on the line to initiate a major shift in policy. He had done this before, as in his espousal of the Great Leap Forward in 1957. When that effort suffered severe reverses —in part because of disastrous crop failures caused by drought and floods—Mao had given up much of the leadership function to Liu Shaoqi and his associates, who included Deng Xiaoping. In 1966 Mao called for a campaign to "bombard the headquarters," to shake up the Party and governmental structure, and to change fundamental priorities.

These central issues of the Cultural Revolution were exemplified, and applied to medicine, in a directive issued by Mao on June 26, 1965, one of the opening statements of the Cultural Revolution. In this message, cited to us repeatedly in the early 1970s as the "June 26th Directive," Mao criticized the Ministry of Public Health for primarily providing care for the urban population while neglecting the needs of the rural population:

> Tell the Ministry of Public Health that it only works for fifteen percent of the total population of the country and that this fifteen percent is mainly composed of gentlemen, while the broad masses of the peasants do not get any medical treatment. First they don't have any doctors; second they don't have any medicine. The Ministry of Public Health is not a Ministry of Public Health for the people, so why not change its name to the Ministry of Urban Health, the Ministry of Gentlemen's Health, or even the Ministry of Urban Gentlemen's Health?[1]

Mao continued with an attack on medical education and aspects of medical practice. He ended his blast against the Ministry with the often quoted phrase, "In medical and health work put the emphasis on the rural areas!"

As a result of the nature of the issues raised during the Cultural Revolution and Mao's explicit attack on the Ministry of Public Health, the health care system was one of the social institutions most profoundly affected by the political upheaval of the late 1960s: medical schools were closed; the administrative apparatus of hospitals and other medical institutions was dismantled; key leaders were attacked and kept under arrest for long periods of time, charged with being "revisionist" or "bourgeois" or with "taking the capitalist road"; many professionals, particularly physicians, were given housekeeping tasks or were sent to "May 7 schools" to be "re-educated"; some physicians and other health workers were relocated to rural areas; and others were organized into medical teams to help train rural medical workers and provide services, and through that process be educated themselves about the lives of the vast majority of the Chinese people, the peasants. Some intellectuals, it has since been reported, were so badly abused, physically and emotionally, that they died or committed suicide. A recent estimate, attributed to "unofficial but usually reliable sources," is that 400,000 people were killed during the Cultural Revolution.[2]

As medical institutions went through the process of "struggle, criticism, and transformation" and began to reorganize in the early 1970s, they reflected the principles that pervaded the other sectors of Chinese society; these principles were an amalgam of tenets adopted by Mao and his followers during the long period of revolution prior to 1949 and those prevalent during the Cultural Revolution. The primary emphasis was on providing services for the "workers, peasants and soldiers," but there was a particularly concerted effort to improve all levels of health care in the countryside.

The Chinese during this period emphasized decentralization and "self-reliance" (*zili gengsheng*), more accurately translated as "regeneration through one's own efforts," rather than a centralized health care system. Communes were encouraged to develop their own health care facilities based largely on their own resources; first-level health care in the cities was placed under neighborhood control—rather than control by the more removed district level—and usually reflected the economic and social nature of the neighborhood. Specialized services were available from the county level in the countryside and from the district level in the urban areas, but, for the most part, primary medical care was organized and supervised at the local level. The Chinese did not request or accept foreign aid for technical improvements in medicine or in other sectors, feeling that they must provide for themselves in order to remain truly independent and develop services that truly met China's needs. Aid was refused even for extraordinary natural disasters such as the 1976 earthquake that centered around the mining city of Tangshan, measured 7.8 on the Richter scale, ruined parts of Peking and Tianjin (Tientsin), killed 242,000, and injured 160,000. In contrast, the southern Italian earthquake of 1980, which killed some 3,000 people, led to an extensive international relief effort.

"Put prevention first" continued as a slogan indicating the emphasis on prevention over treatment. Because of this policy, aspects of health care such as family planning, prenatal care, well-baby care, and immunizations were stressed over the treatment of illness and, as a corollary, primary care was emphasized rather than highly technological medicine.

During this period, as in the fifties and early sixties, the Chinese stressed "mobilizing the mass" as a crucial component of their vast health campaigns. Sanitation was still a key target as it had been since the early fifties. Starting in the late sixties, family planning became another target area, particularly in the cities. To facilitate mobilizing the population to participate in these efforts and to provide primary care where little or none existed, emphasis was placed on the recruitment and training of part-time indigenous workers: the barefoot doctor in the countryside, the Red Medical Worker in the urban neighborhood, and the worker-doctor in the factory. Those selected for these roles, usually by their peers, lived and worked among them and continued to do so after the brief periods of local training. The focus of these health workers was on illness prevention, health education, sanitation, and mobilizing the population to take part in health campaigns. These health workers were not regarded as health professionals but constituted a bridge between the larger population and the professional system.

When medical colleges reopened in the early 1970s the curriculum was cut to three years or at most to three and a half years. Emphasis was placed on teaching the practical rather than the theoretical and students spent a significant period of time in medical school working and learning in the rural areas. The recruitment of workers and peasants into medical school was given high priority, and, in an era in which all grades and examinations were discontinued, medical students were chosen by the units in which they lived and worked on the basis of their political ideology, ability, and physical fitness.

During this period there was an attempt to integrate traditional and Western medicine to a greater degree than had been the practice in the early sixties. While the part-time indigenous health workers used both traditional and Western medicine in their work, they relied heavily on traditional techniques. In the newly reopened medical schools traditional medicine was taught alongside Western medicine. During earlier periods doctors trained in Western medicine had been openly skeptical about the efficacy of traditional medicine; during the early seventies traditional medicine had markedly improved its status. One technique, acupuncture anesthesia, was demonstrated widely to Western visitors; it brought the Chinese considerable publicity and, if not acceptance, at least murmurs of wonderment. The use of herbs and other traditional techniques received considerable attention as well.

There were efforts to reduce the power and prestige of physicians and to encourage health workers to work on a more egalitarian basis. And finally, as in the larger society, the emphasis within medicine was on spiritual rewards rather than on material rewards; the medical worker was expected to "serve the people" and, in doing so, obtain gratification from his or her work.

In sum, the emphasis in health during the early seventies was on deprofessionalization, demystification, decentralization, popular participation, providing care for those who formerly had the least, and on "serving the people."

Urban organization and the provision of human services were also profoundly affected by the Cultural Revolution. After a period of frequently intense criticism of neighborhood cadres (administrators, usually but not always members of the Communist Party) during the late 1960s, revolutionary committees composed of the "three-in-one combination" of Communist Party members, members of the People's Liberation Army, and representatives of the mass were organized at the neighborhood level. As in health, other human services that had previously been under the auspices of the district level of urban government were placed under greater local control as part of the Cultural Revolution effort to involve people in their own governance and in their own services; areas such as health care and day care were therefore brought under the administrative aegis of nonprofessionals at the neighborhood level rather than under the control of professionals at the district level.

In preschool facilities, political consciousness, taught largely through the words of Mao Zedong, was a central priority in the early 1970s; identification with the workers, peasants, and soldiers was stressed through a variety of techniques, including the introduction of manual labor into the curriculum.

Primary, secondary, and higher education stressed equality in an attempt to reduce the "three differences" between town and countryside, between worker and peasant, and between mental and manual labor. Major efforts were made to achieve universal primary education and to expand secondary education, the number of years spent in school was reduced, the material taught simplified, and all forms of what was called "elitist education"—key schools, ability groupings, special schools for the cadres' children—were abolished. Practical teaching and learning was stressed over research, politics over technical expertise (better to be "Red" than "expert"), relatively brief periods of training and periods of manual labor were instituted in order that students would not become "divorced from the masses," and students were encouraged to question the earlier emphasis on grades and examinations.

These changes were heralded in the Chinese press, in cinemas, ballets, and "revolutionary Chinese operas," in materials prepared for foreign readership, and in discussions with foreign visitors to China as the beginning of a new phase in China's revolutionary development. Hardship would be shared equally, elites of prestige, power, or income would be curbed (including freezing of higher-level wages until those with lower wages could catch up), and, in general, through diligent work and sacrifice the standard of living of everyone would rise as production increased. No longer were some to be subjected without surcease to alienating or physically debilitating work while others lived lives of relative ease as administrators or professionals. The slogan of the Shanghai dock workers—"we shall be masters of the docks and not merely slaves to tonnage"—was an example of the rhetoric and the goals of the period.

As we have noted in the introduction, these words—and the concepts they conveyed—echoed throughout China and the world. Perhaps it was possible to modernize in ways that would not leave human debris by the wayside and that would share the benefits equitably as they were obtained.

Yet after a decade of turmoil and experimentation, many of the goals and what were seen as reforms of the Cultural Revolution were reversed. Nineteen seventy-six was a watershed year in the history of modern Chinese politics: Premier Zhou Enlai died early in the year after a long illness; Mao Zedong died on September 9. On October 6 Hua Guofeng, who had been named First Vice-Chairman and Zhou's successor by the Chinese Communist Party Politburo on April 7 of the same year, "overthrew" what came to be called the Gang of Four. This group of leaders, who had accumulated significant political power during the early 1970s, was composed of Mao's widow, Jiang Qing, Wang Hongwen, a young Shanghai Communist Party official who had risen to become Vice-Chairman of the Communist Party, Yao Wenyuan, a Shanghai literary and cultural critic, and Zhang Chunqiao, a leading Shanghai official who was considered the "theorist" of the group. They were subsequently accused of creating disruption and confusion throughout China's economy. It was alleged that during the early 1970s conflict about the primacy of politics versus the need for high productivity was rampant. For example, at the Daqing oil field, once touted as a model industrial economic unit, an "ally" of the Gang claimed that rules that set the hours of work and quality control standards were counterrevolutionary; production is said to have declined seriously at Daqing and many other workplaces as factional disputes developed between those who supported the Gang and those who did not. In an incident which became a celebrated example of the struggle during the early and mid-1970s, the main junction of the Peking-Wuhan railway line was virtually paralyzed by internal conflict, a paralysis that seriously affected the country's economy. The response of the Gang of Four was said to have been "Better a socialist train that's late than a capitalist train that's on time." The Gang were also accused of plotting against Zhou Enlai, of banning memorial articles on him after his death, and of plotting against Deng Xiaoping.[3]

The Gang were said to have undermined China's education by the stress on "Red" rather than "expert." They were also accused of keeping China's cultural activities under their tight control and of becoming the sole judges of what was acceptable in the arts; films, operas, and ballets were either rewritten or shelved and many performers were blacklisted and some imprisoned because they were thought to be opposed to Jiang Qing's control.

And finally the Gang of Four, specifically Yao Wenyuan, were accused of stressing spiritual rather than material rewards and undermining the principle "To Each According to his Work," which Yao claimed was part of "bourgeois ideology."[4] Today the phrase "equalitarianism" is used pejoratively to describe the Gang of Four's policy of equality of wages irrespective of the quality or amount of work done.

Deng Xiaoping, who had functioned as de facto premier during 1975 and was regarded as Zhou's likely successor, was removed for a second time (the first was in the early 1970s) from his Party, government, and military positions during the same April 1976 meeting of the Politburo that installed Hua in power; he was once again rehabilitated and in June 1977 was named to the positions of Vice-Premier, Vice-Chairman of the Party, and Chief-of-Staff of the People's Liberation Army, making him China's prime leader notwithstanding the titular superiority of Hua Guofeng, the leader "chosen" by Mao in his last days.

Since the autumn of 1976 Chinese politics has been characterized, according to one observer, by "a consensus within the leadership to depart from Mao's revolutionary radicalism and to promote the program of 'four modernizations,' i.e., the modernization of industry, agriculture, science and technology, and the military."[5] As part of Deng's consolidation of power and his emphasis on pragmatic modernization programs, he and his supporters have attempted to destroy what they call the "cult" of Mao and to dilute Mao's ideological authority. Recent statements in *Renmin Ribao* (*People's Daily*) have described Mao as a "great Marxist" but as only one of dozens of out-standing Chinese leaders, "including Sun Yat-sen, Confucius and Genghis Khan."[6] In a recent article in the *Liberation Army Daily* a senior Communist Party official evaluated Mao's role over the years. While the late Chairman was charged with having pushed "socialist revolution and socialist construction" too far and too fast, with having followed policies that led to "great disorder" during the Cultural Revolution and with having lost "contact with the day-to-day life of the masses," the article urged that he be judged with "compassion, love and respect." "Defaming Chairman Mao can only demean the party and our socialist motherland," the article continued.[7] In May 1981 Huang Hua, China's Foreign Minister and Deputy Prime Minister, stated that the current consensus of party leaders is that while Mao made mistakes, such as his initiation of the Great Leap Forward of 1957–1958, he was a "great Marxist and a great revolutionary who was the first to combine the universal principles of Marxism with the concrete conditions of the Chinese revolution." The "consensus," according to Mr. Huang, is that Mao's contributions were primary and his mistakes secondary.[8]

Since the spring of 1978, Deng has been promoting a new ideo-logical tenet which is essentially one of pragmatism: "practice is the sole criterion of truth." In essence this means that a policy is correct if it produces positive results. Perhaps the clearest expression of Deng's pragmatic ideology is his now famous remark made in 1962 that he did not care whether a cat was black or white so long as it could catch mice. According to a recent analysis, "Deng's clarion call is to 'seek truth from facts.' In a system in which party and state constitutions have sanctified Marxism–Leninism–Mao Zedong Thought as the guiding ideology, the idea that Deng has been trying to foster is truly icono-clastic and revolutionary." In conjunction with efforts to promote a new ideological framework Deng has attempted to gain control of the main decision-making bodies by purging Maoists and others opposed to his policies. Despite opposition from Hua and others, Deng has been able to purge many of those who had collaborated with the Gang of Four and to consolidate a network of support both at the national and provincial levels. After the Third Central Committee Plenum in

December 1978 it was clear that Deng was the most powerful leader in China and the primary architect of China's modernization policies and programs.[9] In June 1981 Deng's consolidation of power was further realized as Hua was replaced as Chairman of the Chinese Communist Party by Hu Yaobang, a protégé of Deng's, and Deng himself was named Chairman of the Party's Military Commission, which controls the army.[10]

The current phase of China's development strategy stems from the December 1978 meeting of the Communist Party, during which principles of "readjustment" were adopted. This process has been described as "a major readjustment of the economic relations between the state, the collective and the individual." Official statements in 1981 gave the governmental view that China's plan for economic growth developed soon after the fall of the Gang of Four was overly ambitious and that future plans must be more realistic. China is now openly examining its "previous mistakes, backward methods and outmoded beliefs and practices left over from 'feudal' thinking."[11]

The current official goal is to establish priorities among the economic sectors—agriculture to be given first priority, light industry second, and heavy industry third. Economic management is being transferred from administrative units to economic organizations and the role of market forces is being widely debated. Some Chinese economists are suggesting a greater interplay between central planning and market forces in the hope that local initiative will be more greatly stimulated. At the same time there has been a shift toward smaller economic units, such as breaking down what were viewed as relatively large units at the commune and production brigade level, and a more flexible policy that would take into account local strengths and regional differences of climate and natural resources. One consequence of the smaller units and decentralized planning is that some localities will develop faster than others, exacerbating the already existing differences between relatively affluent and poor areas. Some 3,000 enterprises have been given a larger measure of self-management, and it has been reported that the Chinese have examined the Yugoslav system of worker-management.

During the 1976–1977 period there was a startling policy shift toward importing foreign technology, utilizing foreign loans, and developing heavy industry. Since 1978 emphasis has shifted somewhat from the "microchips with everything" plans for modernization toward what appears to be a more realistic and self-reliant approach of modernizing existing enterprises. For instance, one of the most important symbols of the Four Modernizations policy, development of the huge Baoshan Steelworks near Shanghai, was postponed in 1980, after construction had already begun, because of a shortage of foreign currency, inadequate planning, and a lack of raw materials.

With the current stress on material rewards and the raising of incomes of both peasants and workers, increased production of consumer goods and improved housing and other elements of daily living are being emphasized. The proportion of heavy industry to light industry will be altered in favor of light industry. In Shanghai, for example, the emphasis will be on "sectors requiring technical expertise, precision and skills, areas of high technology involving relatively lower consumption of energy, imposing less of a burden on transportation and not requiring massive inputs of raw materials with which the municipality is not well endowed." In contrast, the province of Anhui, which has little industry and is rich in natural resources, will significantly increase its development of heavy industry.[12]

In agriculture, which has been given highest priority in China's most recent modernization plans, the focus is now on mechanizing those areas in which farm machinery can be used to greatest advantage and encouraging further modernization through a combination of state financial assistance and local efforts. To maximize local input into rural development, communes and brigades are being encouraged to raise their own development funds, in part through increasing the output of their local factories. Peasants are being given greater freedom to choose the crops they will grow, and a new agricultural "responsibility system," adopted since Deng Xiaoping's victory at the Party's Third Plenary Session in December 1978, sets responsibility for crop goals and production at far lower levels of social organization—including the household and individual level—than ever before. Intended to raise the peasants' agricultural production by providing individual and family incentives, the new agricultural policy also supports the extension of peasants' private plots and the reopening of free markets in the city and countryside.

Current Chinese development policy has led to an increased emphasis on technical expertise over political consciousness—an emphasis on being "expert" over being "Red." It has led to a new frankness about the extent of the damage due to natural disasters—such as 1980 droughts in Hebei Province and floods in Hubei Province—and requests for foreign aid from the International Red Cross, the United Nations, and Western countries.[13] It has also led to increased foreign trade with the United States, Japan, and other countries and to a markedly increased exchange among scholars between China and the United States and with other countries.

In medicine the new modernization policies have led to new emphases: on upgrading technology wherever possible; on increased efforts in research; on lengthening courses of study for health workers at all levels; on attempts at quality control for all health workers but particularly for barefoot doctors; and, as in the larger society, on emphasizing expertise over politics.

Urban organization has also undergone significant change in recent years. In 1979 neighborhood committees were abolished throughout China and administrative control over most services was moved to the more centralized district level, as it had been prior to the Cultural Revolution. These administrative changes reflect the current concern with technical quality of services rather than with mass participation and neighborhood coordination and control. Cadres from the district level have significant authority within urban neighborhoods and professionals are once again in control over health care and day care.

Preschool facilities focus, as indeed they have since their initial development in revolutionary China, on the care and well-being of the young child. Recently, however, formal learning is being stressed over ideology. This trend is manifested in the children's performances, the stories they hear, their artwork, the markedly decreased amount of time allotted to manual labor, in fact, in all aspects of their daily curriculum.

Current educational policy at the primary, secondary, and tertiary levels is being restructured to strengthen those schools and other aspects of education in which educational strength is already greatest rather than in those in which it is weakest. Recent years have seen a return to grades and examinations, to students divided by ability; a renewed stress on intense study and on gaining admission into college or technical school; and a focus on acquiring skills and knowledge rather than raising political consciousness.

Political events and economic policies have therefore continued to have a significant impact on health and human services in China. In the following chapters we will attempt to describe and analyze those changes in considerable detail while keeping in mind that China is an ever-changing society, the changes frequently occurring faster than the observer's pen can write.

II | Health Care Services

2 | Four Millennia of Medicine

Health Care in China Prior to Liberation

There are two distinct streams of medicine in modern China—the Chinese terms for them are "Chinese medicine" and "Western medicine." Until the seventeenth century the only medicine in China was "Chinese medicine," what is now called by the rest of the world "Chinese traditional medicine." As in other aspects of Chinese thought, external influences and the few innovations brought by foreigners were simply absorbed into the traditional structure.

The march of Chinese medicine to the seventeenth century was, in comparison to other elements of human technical development, an extraordinarily long one. Chinese medicine is probably the world's oldest body of continuous medical knowledge and tradition, having a history of some four thousand years of accumulated empirical observations and abstruse and complex theory. Its earliest surviving treatise, the *Huangdi Neijing* (*The Yellow Emperor's Classic of Internal Medicine*), which is popularly ascribed to an emperor who is believed to have lived in approximately 2500 B.C. (although the book may have been actually committed to writing much later), states many of its current principles.[1] Babylonian and Egyptian medicine may have preceded Chinese medicine, but little or nothing of those traditions remains today.

By virtue of its rich and ancient theoretical base, Chinese traditional medicine, which incorporates both diagnosis and therapy, differs from many other current systems of folk medicine, which are based purely on empirical observations, and differs from systems based on magic, witchcraft, and spiritualism. Diagnostic methods in Chinese medicine include observing and questioning the patient, limited physical examination, and detailed and prolonged pulse-taking. Therapy uses such techniques as medicinal herbs, acupuncture, moxibustion (the application of heat to sites on the skin), breathing and gymnastic exercises, and flexible splinting.

The theoretical concepts of health and disease are based for the most part on a philosophic explanation of nature, on a belief in the unity of man and the universe. The human body—and its life force *qi*—are considered to be constantly influenced by the complementary forces of *yin* and *yang*; if all the forces are in perfect order, in harmony with the year, the season, and the time of day, the human body is in good health. If there is any disharmony, disease may result. Traditional Chinese medical thought, similar in many ways to that of the ancient Greeks and Arabs and indeed of Europe until the nineteenth century, is based on elements as diverse—yet interrelated in complex ways—as a belief in the harmonious relationship between the macrocosm and the microcosm and the careful observation and classification of the properties of natural products.

The nature of the medicine that flourished in China over the millennia permitted a wealth of empirical observations. Among them was the discovery of the circulation of the blood almost 2,000 years before its discovery in the West. The Chinese also discovered the fundamentals of smallpox inoculation (variolation), for the prevention of the more serious, naturally acquired form of the disease, by the beginning of the sixteenth century;[2] from China the technique was brought by Russian doctors to Turkey, and from there to England and the West at the beginning of the eighteenth century. It was not until 1798, some 200 years after the Chinese had started using smallpox inoculations, that Jenner published his observations—learned from a dairymaid—on cowpox inoculation (vaccination) for the prevention of smallpox.

Physicians were first appointed to the courts of the Chinese emperors during the fourth century B.C. The primary responsibility of government physicians attached to the courts was the examination of the numerous personnel of the palace and the early detection of disease; they were also responsible for food control and general hygiene. Thus the Chinese emphasis on prevention is not simply a contemporary phenomenon; traditionally the physician who knew how to prevent disease was more highly respected than one who waited until the patient was sick. There are quotations surviving from the Warring States period (403–221 B.C.) stating that "the most perfect physician cures a disease before it has ever shown itself at all." The great physician Ge Hong wrote about 320 A.D.:

Thus the adept disperses sufferings (physical or mental) before they have begun; and cures diseases before they have made their appearance. He practices his therapy before any untoward signs have manifested themselves, and does not have to pursue what has already happened.[3]

Under the influence of Daoism, which flourished from the second century to the fifth century after the birth of Christ, Chinese physicians continued their emphasis on prevention through their concern with aspects of physical exercise, diet, and sexual behavior. Moderation in all aspects of living was thought to be essential; insufficient activity was viewed as being as harmful as overexertion. By the end of the Han dynasty in A.D. 220 the Chinese system of traditional medicine was firmly established; it was the only organized medical system in China for the next 1500 years and remained the only medical care available for the vast majority of the Chinese people until after Liberation in 1949.

In addition to specific aspects of theory and techniques of traditional Chinese medicine, the practice of medicine in pre-seventeenth-century China led to the formulation of a series of principles, a number of which continue to influence medicine in China today. These included *Treatment of female patients*: Doctors were greatly influenced, as were the rest of the population, by Mencius' precept that "men and women, in giving and receiving, must not touch each other." Since the female patient could not expose any part of her body to, or be palpated by, a male physician, a female doll was often used as an adjunct to the examination. Female patients in current China, particularly in rural areas, are said to still prefer female physicians. *An emphasis on public service*: Many of the prominent physicians in ancient China were either retired government officers or scholars who had failed in the Imperial examinations. They were said to have provided many free services and to have eschewed large financial return. *Honor to the physician*: Patients used to present wooden boards with complimentary inscriptions as an expression of appreciation to doctors who had treated them successfully. The custom also proclaimed the skill of the doctor to other patients suffering from similar diseases. *Secret prescriptions*: The dispensing of secret prescriptions was not only considered ethical, it was deemed an honor—and more effective for the patient—for the physician to know a secret formula. *Differentiation of patients by class*: The physique of a noble was considered delicate and that of a commoner tough, and they were therefore to be treated differently. Physicians were sometimes classified into two groups, one specialized in treating those of high rank, and the other, the common people. *Just desserts*: It was generally believed that disease and misery were a retribution for past sins while health and happiness were rewards for past virtues.[4]

The last belief was associated with patients' use of medical practices and practitioners that were not part of the formal Chinese medicine tradition but were based on magic and witchcraft. These beliefs have extended into the modern era and have interfered with the use of other medical techniques. The Communist Party's policies in the 1930s and later, while encouraging formal traditional Chinese medicine, discouraged medical magic and witchcraft.[5]

The first Jesuit missionaries began arriving in China at the beginning of the seventeenth century. While this marks the beginning of a new period of medicine in China, penetration of China by Jesuit medicine was limited. Most books imported or written by Jesuits in China were not disseminated to Chinese physicians during the Qing

(Ch'ing) dynasty (1644–1912), allegedly because the Manchu emperor felt the introduction of foreign medicine might "confuse the people."

With the introduction of Western medicine to China, which began in earnest with the missionary efforts of the nineteenth century, there arose great conflicts between the practitioners of the two schools. On one side, stories were spread about "evil practices" of Western doctors; on the other, traditional medicine was condemned as false and superstitious. The Chinese people were often torn between their faith in traditional medicine and the evidence of the efficacy of Western practices, particularly in surgery and obstetrics. In the cities, while the status and prestige of Western doctors increased relative to that of traditional doctors, there were far too few of them to meet the needs of people, particularly the poor. In the rural areas, except for major provincial towns, Western-type medicine was almost nonexistent.

Schools of Western medicine were established in China during the late nineteenth century and the early decades of the twentieth. The first was established in Tianjin in 1881 by a Scottish physician, John Kenneth MacKenzie, and during the next thirty years several other medical schools were founded under the auspices of foreign governments. By 1913 there were approximately 500 Chinese students studying Western medicine in China under the auspices of foreign powers and only a relatively small number of Westerners practicing medicine in China.

The outbreak of pneumonic plague in Manchuria in 1911 significantly advanced the cause of Western medicine in China. During the five-month duration of the disease 60,000 people died. Because they did not know how to protect themselves, there was a 50 percent mortality rate among practitioners of Chinese medicine, while among practitioners of Western medicine the rate was only 2 percent. Wu Liande, a physician who helped fight the epidemic, later wrote that this outbreak of plague

> definitely laid the foundation for systematic public health work in China. Those in authority from the Emperor downwards, who had formerly pledged their faith to old-fashioned medicine, now acknowledged that its methods were powerless against such severe

outbreaks. They were thus compelled to entrust the work to modern-trained physicians and to give their consent to drastic measures, such as compulsory house-to-house visitation, segregation of contacts in camps or wagons, and cremation of thousands of corpses which had accumulated at Harbin and elsewhere.[6]

During the same period, with the establishment of the Rockefeller Foundation in 1913, American interest in bringing Western medicine to China increased sharply. At a conference in China early in 1914 Charles Eliot, president emeritus of Harvard, expressed the American academic view of practitioners of traditional Chinese medicine:

They have no knowledge of the practice of scientific medicine and no knowledge of the practice of surgery in the modern sense. The Chinese physician uses various drugs and medicaments compounded of strange materials, employs charms and incantations, and claims occult powers ... but of scientific diagnosis, major surgery, anesthesia and asepsis he knows nothing ... the treatment of disease in the mass of the Chinese population is ignorant, superstitious and almost completely ineffectual.

President Eliot continued, "We find the gift of Western medicine and surgery to the Oriental populations to be one of the most precious things that Western civilization can do for the East."[7]

Following the conference, the first China Medical Commission recommended, among other activities, the establishment of a "strong" medical school in China. The China Medical Board was established by the Rockefeller Foundation to implement this program. The Union Medical College in Peking was purchased, and in 1916 the second China Medical Commission recommended that admission standards to the new medical school, named the Peking Union Medical College (PUMC), should closely approximate those of the leading American medical schools. Despite the desperate need for physicians, the decision was made to train relatively few academically excellent physicians who would then become the teachers and leaders of medical care and research in China.

Bertrand Russell, who visited Peking in 1920 and saw and praised the architecture of the new college, an extremely costly but harmonious blend of the traditional and the utilitarian, was, however, less than totally enthusiastic about the American medical effort:

> Although the educational work of the Americans in China is on the whole admirable, nothing directed by foreigners can adequately satisfy the needs of the country. The Chinese have a civilization and a national temperament in many ways superior to those of white men. A few Europeans ultimately discover this, but Americans never do. They remain always missionaries—not of Christianity, though they often think that is what they are preaching, but of Americanism.[8]

The PUMC was to become a center of excellence in a country racked by poverty, hunger, disease, and eventually war. While the teaching and research were distinguished in many departments in both the clinical and basic sciences, the work in public health is particularly noteworthy. John B. Grant, born in China of Canadian parents and educated in Canada and the United States, began to develop a program in public health at PUMC when the college was opened. There were essentially no national or municipal health services in China, and Grant attempted to develop a community-based public health program, establishing an experimental health center in Peking supported jointly by PUMC and the municipality. A program in maternal and child health, which included the training of midwives, operated out of the health center. There was a desperate need for such a program, since, while there were an estimated 200,000 untrained midwives in China during the mid-1920s, there were only 500 trained midwives. A school health program was also developed stressing immunization, sanitation, and health education.

Perhaps the most impressive aspect of Grant's public health work at PUMC was the effort to develop a rural health program in Tingxian (Ting County), 100 miles outside Peking. Village health workers were trained to work with the peasants in the areas of immunization, first aid, the registration of births and deaths, health education, and the treatment of minor ailments. A physician was available at a district health station for referrals and the training of the village health workers. While this program was in some ways a forerunner of the present-day Chinese rural health network, it had little impact because of the political structure of the time and the poverty under which people lived. Nevertheless, some of its elements were nearly twenty years and a revolution ahead of their time for China and untold decades ahead of other developing countries.[9] But this was the exception at PUMC, which was a frank attempt to transplant an elitist copy of the Johns Hopkins Medical School into China, taught its students in English rather than Chinese, and from 1924 to 1942 contributed a total of 313 graduates to meet China's overwhelming needs.

There is common agreement that during the 1930s and 1940s, the state of health of the vast majority of the Chinese people was extremely poor and the health services provided for them were grossly inadequate. The people of China during that period suffered the consequences of widespread poverty, inadequate nutrition, poor sanitation, continuing war, and rampant disease. The death rate was estimated at about twenty-eight deaths annually per 1,000 population, one of the world's highest. The infant mortality rate was about 200 deaths under one year of age per 1,000 live births; in other words, one of every five babies born died in its first year of life.

Most deaths in China were due to infectious diseases, usually complicated by some form of malnutrition. Prevalent infectious diseases included bacterial illnesses such as cholera, diphtheria, gonorrhea, leprosy, meningococcal meningitis, plague, relapsing fever, syphilis, tetanus, tuberculosis, typhoid fever, and typhus; viral illnesses such as Japanese B encephalitis and smallpox; chlamydial illnesses such as trachoma; and parasitic illnesses such as ancylostomiasis (hookworm disease), clonorchiasis, filariasis, visceral leishmaniasis (kala azar), malaria, paragonimiasis, and schistosomiasis. Nutritional illnesses included most known forms of total calorie, protein, and specific vitamin deficiencies, including beriberi, pellagra, and scurvy. "Malnutrition" was often a euphemism for gross starvation.[10]

Preventive medicine was essentially nonexistent in most of China. Therapeutic medicine of the modern scientific type was almost completely unavailable in the rural areas—where 85 percent of China's people lived—and for most poor urban dwellers. The number of physicians in China in 1949 who were trained in Western medicine has been estimated at no more than 40,000, approximately one doctor for every 15,000 people in China at that time, and was probably considerably less.[11] Most of these were either doctors from Western countries, usually missionaries, or doctors trained in schools in China supported and directed from abroad; the doctors were mainly concentrated in the cities of eastern China.

Nurses and other types of health workers were in even shorter supply, and the minimal efforts in the 1930s to train new types of health workers to meet the needs of China's rural population were largely controlled from abroad, usually poorly supported by the people they were supposed to serve and poorly integrated with their lives and needs.

The bulk of the medical care available to the Chinese people was therefore provided by the roughly half-million practitioners of traditional medicine, who ranged from poorly educated pill peddlers to well-trained and widely experienced practitioners of the medicine the Chinese had developed over millennia. These practitioners and those who practiced Western medicine remained deeply mistrustful of each other and blocked each other's efforts in many ways.

Probably most important of all, three fourths of the Chinese people were said to be illiterate. Cycles of flood and drought kept most of the people starving or, at the least, undernourished. And the limited resources that did exist were maldistributed, so that a few lived in comfort and the vast majority lived a life of grinding poverty. Feelings of powerlessness and hopelessness were widespread; individual efforts were of little avail, and community efforts were almost impossible to organize.

Health Care from Liberation to the Cultural Revolution

Experiments in meeting the overwhelming health needs were started during the 1930s and 1940s by Mao Zedong and the People's Liberation Army, first in the Jiangxi Soviet and then, after the Long March, in the areas around Yan'an (Yenan) in Shaanxi Province. Mao and his colleagues gave health care relatively high priority, both as a method of organizing the peasants and winning them to the Communist side and as a method of maintaining the strength of their forces. Their efforts included mobilizing the people to educate themselves and encouraging them individually and collectively to provide their own health care and medical care services. It was during this period that a few physicians from abroad, such as Norman Bethune from Canada and George Hatem (Ma Haide) from the United States, joined Mao's forces and provided direct services, training, and valuable advice.

When the Communist government assumed power over the entire country (with the exception of Taiwan) in 1949, high priority was given to the establishment of an efficient health care system organized so as to cover the entire population. Four basic guidelines for the organization of medical care were enunciated at the People's Republic of China's first National Health Congress in August 1950:

1. Medicine should serve the workers, peasants and soldiers

2. Preventive medicine should take precedence over therapeutic medicine

3. Chinese traditional medicine should be integrated with Western scientific medicine

4. Health work should be combined with mass movements

Some of the efforts of the 1950s and early 1960s were in large measure based on models from other countries, particularly the Soviet Union, which provided a large amount of technical assistance to China during this period. A number of new medical schools were established, some of the older ones were moved from the cities of the east coast to areas of even greater need further west, and class size was vastly expanded. "Higher" medical education usually consisted of six years, following the completion of some twelve years of previous education, although some schools accepted students with less previous schooling and were said to graduate them after only four or five years of medical education. One school, the China Medical College, located in buildings of and employing much of the faculty of the former Peking Union

Medical College, had an eight-year curriculum and was devoted to the training of teachers and researchers.

These efforts produced a remarkably large number of "higher" medical graduates, including stomatologists, pharmacologists, and public-health specialists as well as physicians. It has been estimated that more than 100,000 doctors were trained over fifteen years, an increase of over 250 percent. But by 1965 China's population had increased to about 700 million, and the doctor/population ratio was still less than one per 5,000 people compared to more than one per 1,000 in the industrialized countries at that time (see Table 1).

At the same time large numbers of "middle" medical schools were established to train assistant doctors (modeled largely on the Soviet *feldshers*—medical workers similar in many ways to military corpsmen[12]), nurses, midwives, pharmacists, technicians, and sanitarians. These schools accepted students after nine or ten years of schooling and had a curriculum of two to three years. It has been estimated that some 170,000 assistant doctors, 185,000 nurses, 40,000 midwives, and 100,000 pharmacists were trained (see Table 2).

During the period from 1949 to 1965 the number of hospital beds increased from approximately 84,000 (one for every 6,500 people) to approximately 650,000 (one for every 1,200 people) (see Table 3). This was still far less than the ratio of approximately one hospital bed for every 100 people in technologically developed countries, but considerably higher than in other countries at China's level of technological development. In 1965, India, for example, had one bed for every 1,600 people.

In addition to these efforts to rapidly produce many more professional health workers and health facilities, people in the community were mobilized to perform health-related tasks themselves. A large-scale attack was made on illiteracy and superstition. By means of mass campaigns, people were organized so as to accomplish together what they could not do individually. One of the best-known of these campaigns (which were often called the Great Patriotic Health Campaigns)

Table 1
Western-Style Physicians, 1949–1980*

Year	Physicians	Doctor-Population Ratio
1950	41,000	1:15,000
1957	74,000	1: 9,000
1965	150,000†	1: 5,000†
1978	359,000	1: 2,700
1979	395,000	1: 2,400
1980	447,000	1: 2,200

†Estimated.

Table 2
"Professional Medical Workers," 1949–1980*

Year	Higher Level	Middle Level	Lower Level	Tradi-tional	Total
1950	41,000	107,000	n.a.	n.a.	780,000
1957	74,000	300,000†	1,000,000†	5,00,000†	1,908,000
1965	150,000†	500,000†	n.a.	n.a.	n.a.
1978	391,000	1,065,000	663,000	346,000	2,464,000
1979	436,000	1,108,000	737,000	359,000	2,642,000
1980	502,000	1,174,000	753,000	369,000	2,798,000

†Estimated.

More detailed data for 1978 to 1980 are presented in Appendix A; subtotals may not add to totals because of rounding.

Sources for Table 1 and Table 2

Data for 1950 and 1957 from Ten Great Years.[13]

Data for 1965 estimated by Leo Orleans and Chu-yuan Cheng.[14]

Data for 1978 to 1980 provided by the Chinese Ministry of Public Health.[15]

Table 3
Hospitals, 1949–1980*

Year	Hospitals	Hospital Beds	Hospital Bed-Population Ratio
1949	2,600†	84,000	1:6500
1957	5,000†	364,000	1:1800
1965	n.a.	650,000†	1:1200†
1978	64,421	1,856,000	1: 516
1979	65,009	1,932,000	1: 502
1980	n.a.	1,982,000	1: 496

†Estimated

Sources for Table 3

Data for 1949 and 1957 from Ten Great Years.[16]
Data for 1965 estimated by Chinese physicians visiting Canada, 1971.[17]
Data for 1978 and 1979 from China Encyclopedia Yearbook, 1980.[18]
Data for 1980 from Beijing Review.[19]

was the one aimed at eliminating the "four pests," originally identified in some areas—but not all—as flies, mosquitos, rats, and grain-eating sparrows. When the elimination of sparrows appeared likely to produce serious ecological problems, bedbugs (and in some areas lice or cockroaches) were substituted as targets. People were also encouraged to build sanitation facilities to keep their neighborhoods clean.

Campaigns against specific diseases were also mounted. Thousands of people were trained in short courses to recognize the symptoms and signs of venereal disease, encourage treatment, and administer antibiotics when necessary. At the same time the brothels were closed or turned into small factories, and the prostitutes were treated and then retrained or sent back to their homes in the countryside. There were also mass campaigns against opium use. Epidemic-prevention centers were established to conduct massive immunization campaigns and to educate people in sanitation and other disease-prevention techniques.

Another example of the use of mass organization in health was the campaign against schistosomiasis, a parasitic illness acquired from working barefoot in contaminated water. Part of the development of the parasite takes place in snails, hence the term "snail fever." This campaign was based, according to Joshua Horn, a British surgeon who worked in China for fifteen years, on the concept of the "mass line"— "the conviction that the ordinary people possess great strength and wisdom and that when their initiative is given full play they can accomplish miracles." [20]

The idea behind the antischistosomiasis program was not only to recruit the people to do the work but also to mobilize their enthusiasm and initiative so that they would fight the disease. The antischistosomiasis effort is particularly illustrative of mass participation, since it mobilized the population in several directions: to move against the snails, cooperate in case finding and treatment, and improve environmental sanitation.

In all these health campaigns it was repeatedly stressed that health is important not only for the individual's well-being but also for that of the family, the community, and the country as a whole. The basic concept of the mass health campaign is said to be the recognition of a problem important to large numbers of people, the analysis of the problem and recommendation of solutions by technical and political leaders, and then—most important—the thorough discussion of the analysis and recommended solutions with the people so that they can fully accept them as their own.

In therapeutic medicine, modern technology was being introduced, but change was relatively slow and was concentrated in the urban areas. A campaign to integrate Chinese medicine with Western medicine was initiated and designed to: (1) make full use of those elements of Chinese medicine that were found effective; (2) provide greater acceptance of Western techniques among those, particularly in the rural areas, who mistrusted them; and (3) efficiently employ the large numbers of practitioners of Chinese medicine. The campaign met with some success, but there was said still to be considerable resistance on both sides and integration was slow and incomplete. [21]

Health Policy and Its Results, 1949–1965

In sum, since 1949 health policy in China has reflected the dominant political ideology of the period. This has always been true, in China as in other countries, but is seen with extraordinary clarity in China. During the first five years after Liberation, in part because the Communist Party lacked trained people, physicians and professionals in the Ministry of Public Health largely shaped health policy. From 1955 through 1957 the Chinese leadership attempted to deal with the problem of "how to produce fundamental social change and simultaneously obtain the cooperation of the professionals necessary to make any such effort successful."[22] The Ministry of Public Health was thought to be "divorced from Party leadership" and was attacked with increasing intensity, particularly for opposing traditional medicine. Consequently, party leaders were gradually placed in the Ministry and certain policy-making decisions were removed from the Ministry's authority.

The late 1950s was a period of further division between the Party and the Ministry of Public Health. While the Ministry was frequently criticized for deemphasizing rural health care, Mao's concern about the discrepancy between life in the cities and living conditions in the countryside and his concern about the consequent alienation of the peasants led to an attempt at rapid transformation of the rural areas. During the period of the Great Leap Forward (1957–1958), the responsibility for health care was further fragmented by the development of people's communes. Commune clinics that were almost completely independent of the Ministry (unlike those of the post–Cultural Revolution period) were organized and mass mobilization efforts were often under Party control. Mao's analysis of health policy focused on the undersupply and underutilization of health resources; the analysis of the Ministry of Public Health was that the problem was excess demand and constricting resources under its control.[23] Because decision-making had been fragmented during the Great Leap Forward in health and in other areas, program coordination had become all but impossible.

The economic difficulties of the late 1950s resulted in diminished decision-making power over health policy by the political sector and by commune leadership. During the early sixties, therefore, the Ministry of Public Health once again became the primary decision-making body vis-à-vis health issues and during this period the emphasis once again was on "quality" care and on urban services.

These policy shifts seemed major to many within China, and to many outside, but in retrospect they were relatively modest adjustments in a fundamental policy that emphasized preventive medicine and integrated development of health care with economic and social development. The results of these fifteen years of effort were extraordinary. Diseases such as smallpox, cholera, typhus, and plague were completely eliminated. Diseases such as malaria, filariasis, tuberculosis, trachoma, schistosomiasis, and ancylostomiasis were still not under full control, although their prevalence was markedly reduced. In short, the successes in the prevention of infectious disease over a span of only one generation were truly monumental, but there was still much preventable infectious disease, particularly in the rural areas.

Medical care was increasingly provided publicly rather than privately, in organized primary care services, and vigorous attempts were made to induce physicians and other health workers to practice in rural areas. All medical students graduating in 1963, for example, were said to have been assigned to the countryside. But there was still considerable resistance by graduates of "higher" medical schools to practicing in the rural areas. Despite the massive efforts, medical workers and hospitals were still largely concentrated in the cities. In Guangdong Province, for example, in 1967 two thirds of the hospital beds, 70 to 80 percent of government funds, and 60 percent of high-level medical personnel were assigned to the cities, in which some 20 percent of the province's people lived. The ratio of doctors to population was 1:600 in Guangzhou, the provincial capital, compared with 1:10,000 in the rural areas.[24] In short, after extraordinary achievements over fifteen years, particularly in public health, in the mid-1960s much of the huge rural population still lacked access to basic medical care and much of the urban population still lacked adequate modern medical care.

3 | Shoes for the Barefoot Doctor?

In discussions of health and medical care services in most societies it is useful to make a relatively sharp distinction between "health" services—those devoted to health promotion and disease prevention—and "medical" services—those devoted to the care of those who have become ill or suspect they are ill. It is also useful in most societies to distinguish between "personal" services—those provided to an individual, such as counseling on cessation of smoking or treatment for cancer—and "community" services—such as mass educational campaigns against smoking and public screening programs for cancer. In many societies, such as the United States, "medical" and "personal" services are largely in the private sector and "health" and "community" services are largely in the public sector.

In China such distinctions are much harder to make. Not only are all services—personal as well as community—almost entirely in the public sector but health promotion and disease prevention are closely intertwined with medical care for illness. The barefoot doctor, for example, provides both treatment for the disease or injury of individuals and personal and community preventive services.

Nonetheless, since distinctions must be made to permit clear organization of the material for presentation, we have—somewhat arbitrarily—included in this chapter services that are predominantly personal and therapeutic in nature (and the other work closely intertwined with them) and have left for the next chapter services that are predominantly community-based and preventive in nature (and their associated programs). In this chapter, therefore, we will cover rural and urban medical care and health care services, traditional medicine, and the training of medical care personnel; in chapter four we will cover occupational and environmental health services, the family planning program, and the health statistics of China.

Medical Practice in the Rural Areas

Some roughly 850 million of China's one billion people live in its rural areas, by far the largest rural population of any nation in the world, almost double the rural population of India, the second largest. The people are, moreover, most unevenly distributed. The population is extremely sparse in China's western mountains and deserts, where 4 percent of its people live on 50 percent of its land mass, and extremely dense—even in the agricultural areas—in the fertile river valleys of eastern China.

China has worked hard to keep its population out of its cities. In 1949 eleven percent of China's people lived in urban areas. Because of urban migration during the People's Republic's first decade, described in chapter five, by 1957 over 15 percent of the population lived in cities and towns. Stricter controls on urban migration, attempts at rustification of urban young people during the Cultural Revolution, and a higher birth rate in the countryside than in the cities (with death rates falling comparably in both areas) have led to a greater gain of rural population than of urban population since 1957. The official 1978 estimate was 12.5 percent urban; in 1979 it was 13.2 percent urban, perhaps in part because of a return of rusticated youth to the cities.[1]

Rural areas are in general far poorer than the urban areas. The old exploitative landlord system is of course gone, but there remains considerable variation in income from region to region based on such factors as the productivity of the land, the amount of livestock, and population density.

China's countryside is divided into communes, which are economic, political, social, and paramilitary units. There is common ownership of land except for small private plots for each family. Communes range in size from approximately 10,000 to 60,000 people. The smallest subdivision of the commune is the "production team," with a membership of several hundred people. The team leadership is responsible for the overall planning of the team's work. People on the same production team live close to one another, usually in small villages, and form the basic social unit in the countryside. Several teams combine to form a "production brigade," which usually has wider responsibility than the team with regard to health, transportation, and, in the north, the grinding and storing of grain. A typical commune is composed of ten to thirty production brigades. The commune is the lowest level of formal state power in the rural areas and is responsible for planning, education, health and social services, and the operation of small factories that produce goods for its members and for outside distribution.

As part of the Cultural Revolution effort to deprofessionalize and decentralize aspects of the health care system and to provide care for rural residents, large numbers of peasants were trained to provide elements of environmental sanitation, health education, preventive medicine, first aid, and primary medical care while continuing their farmwork. These peasant health workers came to be known as "barefoot doctors" in the rural areas of Shanghai, where much agricultural work is done barefoot in the rice paddies. Although barefoot doctors actually wore shoes most of the time, especially while performing their medical tasks, the term is used to emphasize the fact that these health workers did not become part of the professional health care system but instead remained peasants who performed their medical work together with their agricultural tasks.[2]

This was not the first effort to train such health workers in China. For example, in 1958, as part of the Great Leap Forward, physicians in Shanghai organized themselves to go to nearby rural areas ". . . where, in cooperation with the clinics of the people's communes, they trained in short-term classes and through practice, large numbers of health workers who did not divorce themselves from production. Figures for June 1960 show that there were over 3,900 such health workers in the more than 2,500 production brigades of the ten counties under the Shanghai municipality."[3]

During the period 1961–1965 there was said to have been a cessation of training and a reduction in the number of such health workers. A report, criticized during the Cultural Revolution as "revisionist," "counterrevolutionary," and "malicious," was issued condemning the role of the health workers in the production brigades and suggesting that it would be better if they dropped their medical work and devoted themselves to agricultural tasks. The 3,900 health workers in the Shanghai counties were therefore reduced in number to just over 300. In the months immediately preceding the Cultural Revolution the training of rural health workers was apparently resumed, and by the time Mao Zedong issued his "June 26th Directive" in 1965 the number of health workers in production brigades of the Shanghai counties had increased to more than 2,300.

The training of barefoot doctors began in earnest following Mao's directive. By 1968 there were 4,500 barefoot doctors in the Shanghai countryside who themselves had trained more than 29,000 peasants as auxiliary "health workers" for the production teams. In 1971 we were told that the 2,724 production brigades in the rural counties of the Shanghai municipality were served by 7,702 barefoot doctors.

In the early 1970s, barefoot doctors performed a wide variety of tasks. In the area of environmental sanitation, the barefoot doctor had responsibility for, among other things, the proper disposal and later use of human feces as fertilizer, for the purity of drinking water, and for the control of and campaigns against "pests." Many of the sanitation tasks were usually carried out during lunch hours and "spare time" by health aides whom the barefoot doctors trained and supervised.

Health education, the provision of primary medical care and preventive measures such as immunizations were other important tasks of barefoot doctors. They were also readily available to deal with medical emergencies, since they often worked in the fields with their patients and lived among them. They were said to be skilled in first aid and in the treatment of "minor and common illnesses." Perhaps most important, their fellow workers knew them well and trusted them.

The initial training of the barefoot doctors took place locally for a period which ranged from three to six months, usually either in the commune or county hospital. Subsequent continuing supervision and additional training periods were used to improve their knowledge and skills. Barefoot doctors were encouraged to use a wide range of both traditional Chinese and Western medicines, and some had become skilled enough to perform limited forms of major surgery.

Barefoot doctors were selected by members of the production brigades they were to serve and were trained and supervised locally. As a result, there was a great range of capabilities and skills. The barefoot doctors usually worked in health stations at the production brigade level, but did much of their work, both medical and agricultural, with their fellow members of the production team. Their income was generally determined in the same way as that of the other peasants in the commune, each peasant's earnings depending on the total income of the brigade and the number of "work points" that the individual collects. Barefoot doctors receive work points for health work just as they would for agricultural work. The work points assigned are generally at the high end of the scale, equivalent to the points received by peasants performing heavy physical labor; on a scale of 1 to 10 points, the barefoot doctors are usually awarded 8 to 10 points for their work.[4]

During the period before the Cultural Revolution, a limited number of urban health workers had been organized in mobile health teams and had traveled the countryside providing services and training. With the advent of the Cultural Revolution, most urban medical workers were required to play a role in these teams or in long-term assignment to a particular rural site, and a rotation system was organized so that at any given time about one third of urban health workers were serving outside the cities. They were there not only to provide services for those living in the countryside but also, it was said, to be themselves "reeducated" by the experience.

In addition to services within the production team and in the brigade health stations, rural medical care was provided by professionally trained personnel in commune and county hospitals. Facilities, particularly in the commune hospitals, were spartan and the level of technology was low, not only when compared to that of industrialized societies but also in comparison to the technology in urban hospitals in China.

During the mid-1970s, and particularly after the fall of the Gang of Four, there began to be considerable criticism of the barefoot doctors. Their training was said to be uneven, their supervision sometimes inadequate, and their practice, at times, incompetent. Examples of mistakes made by barefoot doctors appeared in the Chinese press and were described in interviews with foreign visitors. The examples included instances of inadequate treatment, such as the death of an elderly woman with lobar pneumonia following a barefoot doctor's misdiagnosis of a common cold. Other examples suggested that some barefoot doctors went beyond the limits of their technical knowledge and skills and treated patients in ways that were inappropriate. Some of the current criticism of the Gang of Four period goes even further. It suggests that the barefoot doctors were used as a political weapon, in an attempt to give them control over the entire rural health care system and to permit them to practice medicine as physicians.

While some, with the clear support of Mao, strongly defended the barefoot doctors as one of the valuable "newborn things" of the Cultural Revolution, Deng Xiaoping emphasized how much further they had to improve: "Barefoot doctors cannot reach heaven at a single bound... The barefoot doctors have only just begun; their knowledge is slight. They can only treat a few common sicknesses. After some years, they will put on straw shoes; that is, their knowledge will have grown. A few years more, and they will wear cloth shoes." Deng is said to have symbolically walked out of a screening of a film produced during the Cultural Revolution that showed, he felt, a barefoot doctor going well beyond his training.[5]

In the late 1970s, in keeping with the Chinese drive to improve technical quality, local departments of public health began to markedly upgrade the training of barefoot doctors, require the demonstration of their knowledge through examinations, define their role more narrowly, reduce their numbers, increase their supervision by more extensively trained medical personnel, and to some extent centralize the structure in which they work. What has not changed, however, is the basic economic structure of the barefoot doctors' payment or the basic peer relationship (as contrasted with "professional-to-patient" relationship) of barefoot doctors with the members of the production brigade of which they are a part.

Generalization about these changes is difficult, just as it was difficult to generalize about the barefoot doctors' training and role in the early 1970s. The reasons for the difficulty are many. Because of the emphasis on decentralization, the barefoot doctor pattern varies widely, from province to province, from commune to commune within a province, and even, though far less markedly, from brigade to brigade within a commune. In addition, "rich" brigades and communes have more extensive programs than do "poor" brigades and communes. It is the relatively well off communes that most visitors are taken to see and that are the subject of most of the published reports by the Chinese.

The number of barefoot doctors has diminished since the mid-seventies. Overall, Chinese estimates of the total number of barefoot doctors in China have fallen from 1.8 million in 1975 to approximately 1.5 million in 1980.[6] This appears to be related to the current Chinese emphasis on "quality" rather than "quantity." In the China-Rumania People's Commune outside Peking, for example, the number of barefoot doctors has been reduced from 450 for a population of 46,000 in 1972 to 250 for a population of 48,000 in 1980. According to the commune leaders, "some have become workers, some have gone into the army, some [usually women] have married and moved away, some were promoted to cadres and some went to the university." In Shunyi County, where the population increased slightly from 1971 to 1979 (450,000 to 467,000), the number of professional medical workers almost doubled during the same period (from 676 to 1,175) while the number of barefoot doctors decreased (from 1,400 to 1,200). In 1977 the number of barefoot doctors was still 1,400, so the reduction took place between 1977 and 1979. The reduction was most significant in those production teams with greatest ratios of barefoot doctors to peasants, in which it was felt that there were "too many" barefoot doctors. As in the China-Rumania People's Commune, those who stopped being barefoot doctors included those (largely women) who married and moved to another village, those who became industrial workers, those who went to the university, plus a group that went on to secondary medical schools and medical colleges. In Shunyi County, a total of 300 barefoot doctors during the decade went to secondary medical school or medical college and are no longer working at the production brigade or production team level.

Training beginning in 1977 became longer and more theoretically based, differing considerably from the three months of initial training in the commune hospital that had existed early in the decade. New barefoot doctors now, in the communes we visited, have at least six months of initial training, some or even all of it at the county hospital rather than the commune hospital. Formal—albeit limited—study of pre-clinical sciences such as microbiology and pharmacology is now included, in contrast to the more practical clinical emphasis of the training earlier in the decade.

Continuing education of barefoot doctors was also expanded during the decade. They began to take more specialized courses in traditional and Western medicine, in basic surgery, and in other specific areas within the broad field of primary care. These courses are given at the commune hospital or at the county hospital, usually over a period of three months. Yexian (Ye County) in Shandong Province has in addition set up a school for the advanced training of barefoot doctors, with courses lasting as long as a year. Barefoot doctors typically leave their production teams during these training periods and live at the training site; it is common for the short courses to be given at times of less intense agricultural activity. The barefoot doctors continue to be paid in the usual way during the training period, by the award of work points by their production team.

Both initial and continuing education courses are given by doctors regularly assigned to the commune and county hospitals and by doctors from urban hospitals who travel to these sites on a temporary basis to provide clinical care, consultation, and training. Barefoot doctors themselves, it appears, play a limited role as teachers. More recently, there is less assignment of urban health workers to the countryside on either a fixed basis or on mobile medical teams. More of the training, as well as more of the clinical work, is therefore provided by doctors permanently assigned on a salaried basis to the commune.

Formal, areawide examinations for barefoot doctors began to be administered in 1979 in the Shanghai and Peking municipalities. During the summer of 1979 "nearly 10,000 barefoot doctors from Peking's 14 rural counties and suburban districts took part in an examination given by the city's Bureau of Public Health to check on their professional ability."[7] A copy of the Peking examination was given to us during our visit to China in 1980 and a translation is given in Appendix B. The exam includes material on the examination and treatment of patients with illnesses such as rickets, acute gastroenteritis, and acute appendicitis, and on preventive practices such as immunization and safe water supply. Aspects of both traditional Chinese medicine and Western medicine are included, with questions on physiology and pathology from the Western viewpoint and on the theories of diagnosis and treatment in traditional medicine. The Peking Bureau of Public Health provides syllabuses and other materials to help the barefoot doctors prepare for the examination. Of the barefoot doctors who took the examination in the Peking municipality, 83 percent passed and were granted, according to the official Chinese News Agency, "licenses to practice medicine." More precisely, interviews with barefoot doctors who took the examination and with their teachers—and examination of the licenses themselves—indicate that the licenses identified those who passed as accredited barefoot doctors and did not change their basic role or practice pattern. Those who failed to acquire a passing grade were to receive further training and to be given another chance to pass the exam; they were permitted to continue working on preventive medicine, such as immunization and maternal and child health. If they fail a second time, they will be permanently limited to preventive work or may be assigned to other tasks.

Of the 250 barefoot doctors at the China-Rumania People's Commune, for example, 200 took the exam in August 1979 and of these 186 passed. The fourteen who did not pass were to be given a two-month "refresher course" at the commune hospital before taking the exam again. At the Yangsheng Commune in Shunyi County, barefoot doctors in 1979 took two examinations, at both the county and the commune levels. They were required to pass both sets of examinations in order to receive their barefoot doctor certificates.

In the Shanghai municipality the examination procedure was

apparently more decentralized to the county or commune level. The Bureau of Public Health of one county, for example, provided study outlines with over 300 questions for review. Of the 83 barefoot doctors in the Ma Qiao (Horse Bridge) People's Commune, 56 took the exam in December 1979 and 40 passed it. A second examination was scheduled for summer 1980 for those who did not pass or did not take the first exam. By the end of 1981 barefoot doctors must have passed the examination or they would not be able to see patients independently. The future role for those who do not pass has not yet been decided; one suggestion is that they may become health workers auxiliary to the barefoot doctors.

The production brigade health stations, from which the barefoot doctors work, are the first level of the "three-tiered medical and health network" that serves China's countryside. In the counties of the Shanghai municipalities, peasants' income began to increase sharply in 1981, due, it is said, to the new emphasis on family responsibility, private plots, and private markets. The barefoot doctors' income, still based largely on work points, is beginning to fall significantly behind those of other peasants in their communes. There is now discussion of changing the method of remuneration of the barefoot doctors and even of changing the name to "rural doctor" (*nongcun yisheng*) to reflect their higher level of training and income.

There has also been marked change over the past few years in medical care at the other two levels—the commune and county hospitals. In Shunyi County of the Peking municipality, for example, in 1972 there were 7 commune hospitals and 12 commune "clinics" to serve the county's 19 communes. By 1980 there had only been a very small increase in the county's population but the number of communes had increased to 29. There were now eight "central" commune hospitals, each in charge of hospital care for several communes, and 21 "second level commune hospitals." This appears to be part of an attempt to rationalize the system by structuring a hierarchy of hospitals each of which refers when necessary to the next higher level in a defined pattern. Commune hospitals retain their roles in directing sanitation efforts, promoting family planning and maternal and child health, and "mobilizing and organizing the peasants."

The number of professional medical workers in the county has increased 74 percent, from 676 in 1971 to 1,175 in 1979. Since the county population increased little, the per capita increase from (1.5/1,000 to 2.5/1,000) is also close to 70 percent. Of the specific types of personnel, the number of nurses grew most rapidly, from 65 in 1971 to 143 in 1979, a rise of 120 percent.

As part of the effort to upgrade technological services, the facilities and the personnel of county hospitals are being especially strengthened. The county hospital in Shunyi County illustrates these efforts. In 1972 there were 143 professional medical workers, of whom 43 (30 percent) were doctors and assistant doctors of Western medicine, 5 (3 percent) were doctors and assistant doctors of traditional medicine, 63 (44 percent) were nurses, and 32 (22 percent) were pharmacists and technicians. In 1980 the number of professional medical workers rose to 262, of whom 109 (41 percent) were doctors and assistant doctors of Western medicine, 9 (3 percent) were doctors and assistant doctors of traditional medicine, 87 (33 percent) were nurses, and 57 (22 percent) were pharmacists and technicians. In other words, in the hospital the number of Western medical doctors and assistant doctors rose 133 percent, doctors and assistant doctors of traditional medicine rose 80 percent, nurses rose 38 percent, and pharmacists and technicians rose 78 percent. The major increase in professional staffing was in doctors and assistant doctors, with a marked relative decrease in nurse staffing. Part of the reason for this relative decrease in nurses in the county hospital is that many have been assigned to work in the central commune hospitals. Of the 143 nurses in Shunyi County in 1979, 56 worked outside the county hospital; in 1972 only 2 out of the 65 nurses in the county worked outside the county hospital.

The number of hospital beds in the county changed little during the decade (there was actually a small decrease in 1980 from the 200 beds in 1972 because construction was being done), but 100 new beds were scheduled for completion in 1981. This will conclude with the graduation of 90 new nurses from the secondary medical school located in the hospital; most of the graduates will remain in the county hospital to staff the new beds and relatively few will be assigned outside it.

There have also been recent political changes in the leadership of the hospital. From the late 1960s until 1979 the hospital was run by a revolutionary committee that included representatives of the hospital workers. In 1979 the revolutionary committee was dissolved and replaced in its leadership role by a director, deputy director, and department heads, a return to the pre–Cultural Revolution pattern. Today there are no workers in leadership or decision-making positions. It should be noted that the current director of the hospital had been the chairman of the revolutionary committee, suggesting that even within the revolutionary committee structure the high-level physicians and administrators made the critical decisions.

With regard to the financing of health care in the rural areas, early in the Cultural Revolution a collective yet decentralized approach —called *hezuo yiliao*, "cooperative medical services"—began to be actively advocated. It was later to be identified by the supporters of the Cultural Revolution as one of the two "newborn things" that the Cultural Revolution brought to health care, the other being the bare-foot doctor. The critics of the Cultural Revolution of course claimed that neither concept was new and that both were badly implemented and used for partisan political purposes.

Cooperative medical services are generally set up at the commune or production brigade level. Early in the 1970s when the programs were being developed, commune members had the option to join or not join the system; indeed a few peasants—those still considered to be "class enemies"—were not permitted to join. In recent years, however, if the commune members decide collectively to form a cooperative medical service everyone in the commune must participate.[8]

The annual membership fee for each peasant is determined by the previous year's medical expenses within the commune. If the commune limits expenses, for example, by substituting locally grown herb medicines for more expensive Western medicines or by limiting referral to city hospitals for specialty care, the premiums will be lower. Annual membership fees reported by fifteen communes across China in 1973 ranged from 0.35 to 3.60 yuan per person; the premiums range from less than 1 percent to approximately 3 percent of a family's disposable income. While this is a very low figure for technically developed countries, it is not inconsiderable for people of very low income. It was reported in 1973 that 70 percent of China's 50,000 communes had introduced cooperative medical services.

Some analysts have speculated that one of the reasons all communes in the country still do not have such a system is the financial burden that paying premiums places on commune members.

In addition to the premiums paid directly by peasant families, there are contributions to the support of health services from the production team, commune, and national level. Each production team pays a certain amount of money from its collective welfare fund for each team member subscribing to the cooperative medical service; each commune contributes money from its welfare fund—part of its "public accumulated fund" contributed by production teams—toward the medical services. This system may allow peasants in high-income communes, which accumulate larger welfare funds, to pay smaller individual premiums than do peasants in low-income communes.

The national government attempts to even out some of the inequalities among provinces and communes by allocating health funds to provinces for use in rural areas; the province allocates its funds to the counties and the counties determine the allocation to each commune. There are also subsidies from the urban areas to the rural areas in the form, for example, of mobile medical teams of urban medical workers whose salaries and travel expenses are entirely paid by the urban unit that sent them and, finally, there is the direct support of construction of hospitals and other medical facilities in rural areas by funds from the central government.

Members of the cooperative medical services must still pay an additional fee of 5 to 10 fen for each visit to the health station. This fee helps pay the station's maintenance expenses, excluding the salaries of the barefoot doctors who are paid from production team funds. The registration fee is said to discourage "indiscriminate use" of services. It is reported that during the early days of cooperative medical services, when registration fees were not charged, there were "unnecessary visits and requests for tonic herbs" and some cooperative services "had to be discontinued because of their large deficits."[9]

Visits by peasants to county or city hospitals are in part reimbursed by brigade or commune health funds, but only if the patient is referred by the barefoot doctor or by other commune health care personnel. Some communes pay 50 percent of the costs; others pay fixed amounts with the rest of the expenses paid by the patients themselves. For patients from these communes, a long stay in a city hospital may represent a heavy financial burden.

In reporting on their cooperative medical services in 1974, the revolutionary committee of one region indicated the close connection between the "new creation by the masses" and other political, social, and economic goals:

> Experience has taught both the cadres and the masses of the Changwei Administrative Region that the key to consolidating and developing the cooperative medical service is to adhere to the principles of self-reliance, industry and thrift, and that by merely relying on buying drugs and coveting what is "big" and "foreign," they cannot make their cooperative medical service a success. There is no way but the road of self-reliance.[10]

Overall in China there has been a considerable shift in medical resources toward the rural areas. In 1949 only 25 percent of China's hospital beds were in rural areas and these were of course far less technically adequate than even the technically poor hospitals of the cities. In 1979, China's Minister of Public Health reported, 62 percent of hospital beds were in the rural areas, with a rising technological level.[11] Severe problems of maldistribution of course remain: technical medical care is still considerably less available in the rural areas than in the cities.

Wide differences in medical care resources also exist among provinces and autonomous regions, as shown in Table 1. As expected, the three independent municipalities (Shanghai, Peking, and Tianjin) have higher health care personnel to population ratios and among the highest hospital beds to population ratios. The industrialized Northeast (Heilongjiang, Jilin, and Liaoning Provinces) has considerably higher ratios than the national average, and in general the provinces and regions of the interior south, e.g., Guangxi and Yunnan, are less well provided for than those of the interior north, e.g., Inner Mongolia and Shanxi.

Table 1
Health Care Personnel and Hospital Beds, 1979*

Provinces	Health Care Personnel (per 1000 population)	Hospital Beds (per 1000 population)
Anhui	2.13	1.52
Fujian	2.29	1.84
Gansu	2.48	1.77
Guangdong	2.77	1.83
Guizhou	2.22	1.46
Hebei	2.33	1.70
Heilongjiang	3.99	2.90
Henan	1.79	1.48
Hubei	3.20	2.35
Hunan	2.40	2.21
Jiangsu	2.47	1.93
Jiangxi	2.29	2.09
Jilin	3.75	2.73
Liaoning	4.17	3.13
Qinghai	3.74	2.87
Shaanxi	2.70	1.90
Shandong	2.22	1.60
Shanxi	3.35	2.72
Sichuan	2.37	1.80
Yunnan	2.18	1.87
Zhejiang	2.24	1.58
Autonomous Regions		
Guangxi Zhuang	1.81	1.31
Inner Mongolia	3.54	2.51
Ningxia Hui	3.12	1.95
Tibet	3.61	2.26
Xinjiang Uygur	4.28	3.37
Municipalities		
Peking	8.28	3.08
Shanghai	7.84	4.22
Tianjin	6.22	2.42
Total National	2.37	1.99

*Source: Statistics Section, Statistics and Finance Bureau, Ministry of Health (China Encyclopedia Yearbook, 1980), p. 560.

It is of interest that the relatively isolated, sparsely populated western regions of Xinjiang and Tibet and the province of Qinghai have ratios higher than the national average, evidence of an effort to shift medical resources into them.

Overall, the current distribution—despite the remaining glaring inequities—is said to represent a more considerable equalization of resources—from city to countryside, from north to south, from province to province—than existed in the past.

Medical Practice in the Cities

From the late 1960s through the mid-1970s health care in the urban areas was decentralized to the lowest administrative levels capable of providing the services. By utilizing neighborhood organizations, the place of work, and indigenous paraprofessionals, primary health care was within easy access of the patients and was often provided by health workers with whom the patients lived and worked. Most Chinese cities are divided into districts, districts subdivided into neighborhoods, and neighborhoods, in turn, subdivided into residents' committees. This organizational structure is discussed in greater detail in chapter five. Medical services such as specialty hospitals, sanitation facilities, and "prevention stations" for illnesses such as tuberculosis and mental illness were provided at the district level and were under the administrative aegis of the district Bureau of Public Health. Professional primary care, and much secondary ambulatory care, was provided at neighborhood hospitals by professionally trained medical personnel, and preventive medicine and some primary medical care was provided by street doctors or "Red Medical Workers" at the residents' committee level. All health care at the neighborhood and residents' committee levels was under the administration of the neighborhood revolutionary committee.

Red Medical Workers, almost always women who were not working outside the home, usually received one month of training at the neighborhood hospital, where they learned history-taking and simple physical examination techniques such as blood pressure determination, the uses of a number of Western and herb medicines, and techniques of acupuncture and of intramuscular and subcutaneous injection. Preventive measures such as sanitation, immunization, and birth control techniques were an important part of the curriculum. After their original training, the health workers received continuing in-service training both at their health stations and at the neighborhood hospital.

The Red Medical Workers provided care for patients with "minor illnesses," referred more complicated problems to the neighborhood hospital, and provided follow-up care after a patient had been treated in a hospital. They were paid a modest sum for their work, about fifteen yuan per month, roughly one-third the wages of a beginning factory worker.

A large part of the duties of the Red Medical Worker, under the supervision of the Department of Public Health of the neighborhood hospital, related to sanitation work in the neighborhood—in the summer, campaigns against flies and mosquitoes and attempts to prevent the spread of gastrointestinal disease; in the winter and spring, the prevention of upper respiratory infections. The Public Health Department of the neighborhood hospital also supervised the Red Medical Workers in providing immunizations, which were usually given in the residents' committee health station. The Red Medical Workers often went to the homes to bring the children to the health station for immunization and, if necessary, occasionally gave the immunization in the home.

The Red Medical Workers also had as their responsibility the provision of birth control information. They made periodic visits to all the women of the residents' committee area to encourage the use of contraception. Careful records were kept of the contraceptives used by each woman of childbearing age, defined as the time from marriage to menopause.

Many of the post–Cultural Revolution changes evident in medical practice in the rural areas—increased professionalization, centralization, and technological improvements—are characteristic of health care in the urban areas as well. Responsibility for health care at the most local level in the cities has shifted from the neighborhood revolutionary committees, which were eliminated in 1979, to the Bureaus of Public Health located at the district level. This shift has meant that official responsibility for neighborhood health care now rests with professionals rather than with community activists and local Party leaders, and for these purposes the neighborhood is now called a "subdistrict."

Neighborhood hospitals with fully trained doctors and nurses provide out-patient care for a wide variety of medical problems; problems that the neighborhood hospitals cannot handle are referred to specialized hospitals at the district level.

Urban hospitals at the local level have been considerably upgraded since the fall of the Gang of Four. At the Fengsheng Hospital in the West District of Peking, for example, the number of doctors and nurses has been increased from 58 to 157, new departments have been added, including orthopedics (previously the hospital only had a department of traditional orthopedics), ear-nose-throat, and physical therapy, and facilities now include electrocardiography, electroencephalography, and ultrasound.

The leaders in the hospital claim that the Gang of Four produced "great problems" in their institution. During this period, it is now said, health workers were discouraged from learning new skills and those who tried to study were "persecuted." Intellectuals, known by the epithet "stinking No. 9" (because they were that number on the list of "class enemies"), had to study surreptitiously if they wished to study at all. In addition all workers, it is now reported, were treated the same and paid similar amounts with little distinction made for quality of work or the number of hours worked.

After the arrest of the Gang of Four in 1976, financial management of the hospital was transferred from the neighborhood to the district, responsibilities were more clearly defined, the requirements for each job and the evaluation of each job were spelled out, and rewards were given to the workers based on the fulfillment of their tasks, the quality of their work, and their attendance rate.

Similar changes in a neighborhood hospital are evident in the Chaoyang New Village, a neighborhood of the Putou District of Shanghai. Prior to 1965 the hospital had been managed by the district; during the Cultural Revolution, as part of the emphasis on local control and deprofessionalization, it was placed under the management of the neighborhood revolutionary committee. In 1974 the hospital was returned to the administrative aegis of the district.

The staff of the hospital has been increased significantly: in 1972 there were 57 staff members; in 1980, 141. In 1972 the staff included 25 doctors and assistant doctors and 26 nurses; in 1980 it included 41 doctors and assistant doctors and 39 nurses. In the intervening years seven new departments have been added: electrocardiography, electroencephalography, ultrasound, massage, dentistry, ear-nose-throat, and physical therapy. Since January 1980 the hospital has 30 in-patient beds and four additional beds for observation. Because of the additional staff and equipment, the Chaoyang hospital has also been able to increase the number of daily out-patient visits: in 1972 an average of 400 to 500 patients were seen per day; in 1979 700 to 800 patients were seen per day.

Health care in the streets and lanes, at the level of the residents' committees, is currently provided by "Red Cross Health Workers," comparable to those who were formerly called "street doctors" or "Red Medical Workers." In 1978 the China Red Cross Society, which had been virtually inactive since 1966, began to be revived. By 1980 there were branches in fourteen provinces and municipalities and in the Guangxi Zhuang Autonomous Region. There are now over 110,000 members working in 174 branches in the Peking Red Cross Society and over one million members in the nationwide organization. Since the restructuring of the Red Cross Society, two levels of health workers are engaged in medical work at the residents' committee level: Red Cross "Members" and Red Cross "Health Workers."

Red Cross Health Workers work under the supervision of doctors from the local hospital. Their responsibilities are essentially the same as those of the Red Medical Workers during the Cultural Revolution—treatment of minor illnesses often using traditional techniques such as massage and acupuncture, health education, sanitation, and, of course, a major focus on family planning. Red Cross Members are selected for every courtyard and serve the families who live in that courtyard. Their activities are primarily preventive, but they may also act as aides to others in the system—bringing patients to the hospital or picking up and delivering medication. While the Red Cross Members are volunteers, and therefore unpaid, the Red Cross Health Workers are generally paid a modest stipend. Both groups are composed mainly of women.

In some health stations there appears to be much more professional supervision than during the early 1970s. In the health station of the Wuting Residents' Committee, which is part of the Fengsheng Neighborhood, an assistant doctor and other professionals work daily with the Red Cross Health Workers and "almost every day" a fully trained doctor comes from the Fengsheng Hospital to provide care and supervision. Furthermore, immunization records, which were formerly kept at the health station, were moved to the hospital in 1977. The notices for the immunizations are still sent by the health workers, but the immunizations are now done by physicians either at the hospital or at the health station. Doctors from the hospital also provide ongoing training for the health workers, training which varies according to the seasons. In the summertime, for example, the focus is on gastrointestinal disease, in the winter respiratory disease.

After Liberation in 1949, a widely quoted "instruction" from Mao Zedong—"take good care of the children's health"—and policy decisions in the health service led to special attention to the health of children.[12] Indeed, China's constitution makes a special point of state protection of "the mother and child."[13] Specific objectives developed by the health services to meet this goal include a "search for effective measures to promote the normal growth and development of children, to decrease their morbidity and mortality, and to raise their level of health."[14]

To implement this work, special maternal and child care workers have been trained. Maternal and child health networks are established to coordinate preventive and therapeutic work for this special group. Ambulatory care services at all levels above the residents' committee have special pediatric departments. There are 2,500 specially designated maternal and infant care facilities. In pre–Liberation China there were three children's hospitals, with a total of 173 beds; in 1979 the Ministry of Public Health reported 24 such hospitals, with a total of 4,956 beds.

It is of interest that research on child health has been often combined with the provision of services. For example, surveys conducted by the Institute of Pediatrics of the Chinese Academy of Medical Sciences in 1975—with the Gang of Four in charge of the Ministry of

Health—were described at the time as illustrating a "three-in-one" method for avoiding the "revisionist line of conducting scientific research for the sake of scientific research." The two additional elements combined with the survey examination were the instruction of parents and children on "scientific methods of child care including prevention of childhood diseases" and the "timely treatment of any acute or chronic condition discovered during the physical examination and measurement."[15] The data collected in these and in subsequent surveys are presented in the next chapter.

In the prevention of childhood illnesses, immunization played an important role. During the Cultural Revolution these efforts were the responsibility of the barefoot doctors in the countryside and of the neighborhood health personnel—including the Red Medical Workers—in the cities. The recommended immunization program of the early 1970s included BCG immunization (for the prevention of tuberculosis) for all newborns with boosters for those remaining tuberculin negative at age three and seven; poliomyelitis immunization (with live attenuated virus types I, II and III) at one to three months with boosters at ages one and two; triple immunization (against pertussis [whooping cough], diphtheria, and tetanus) at three to five months with boosters at ages one and three; measles immunization at eight months with a booster at four years; smallpox vaccination at six months with a booster at six years; meningococcal meningitis immunization seasonally; and Japanese B encephalitis immunization seasonally.[16] Although it was clear that there were still difficulties in providing full immunization in the most isolated areas—refrigeration, for example, is necessary for some biological materials and an adequate "cold chain" (transfer from one site of cold storage to another without warming) for delivery was not yet technically feasible because of limited electrification—visitors were shown examples, in both urban and rural areas, of extraordinary completeness of immunizations. The work of the local indigenous health workers and the decentralization of health work were cited as important factors in the completeness of immunization.

In our visits to cities—as well as to rural areas—in 1980, despite considerable technical improvement and professionalization at every level, the health workers at the most local levels still had primary responsibility for health promotion and disease prevention among children and immunization levels remained extremely high.

Referral from the neighborhood hospitals for more specialized care is made to district hospitals or municipal hospitals. In Peking, for example, there are twenty district hospitals and twenty-three municipal hospitals, ten of which have over 500 beds. In addition, there are four highly specialized hospitals run by the Chinese Academy of Medical Sciences (see Appendix C), including:

—The Shoudu (Capital) Hospital, formerly the hospital of the Peking Union Medical College, was called the Fandi (Anti-Imperialist) Hospital from the onset of the Cultural Revolution until 1972. It is a general referral hospital of 550 beds and is responsible for the health care of visitors and diplomatic personnel from Western capitalist countries; James Reston of the *New York Times* had his highly publicized appendectomy there—with acupuncture for postoperative pain relief—in 1971. (Visitors and diplomats from Western socialist countries use the Youyi [Friendship] Hospital, a 600-bed Peking municipal hospital that was called the Fanxiu [Anti-Revisionist] Hospital during the Cultural Revolution.)

—The Fuzhimenwai Hospital, often referred to simply as the Fuwai Hospital, specializes in heart and respiratory illness; 60 to 70 percent of its 350 beds are devoted to cardiology.

—The Ritan Hospital, associated with the Oncology (also translated as "Cancer" or "Tumor") Institute of the Chinese Academy of Medical Sciences, is a specialty hospital for treatment and research in cancer.

Insurance coverage for medical expenses in the cities is of two types. The first, introduced in 1951, is called "public expenses medical insurance" (*gongfei yiliao*). It covers the medical expenses of cadres and students with no contribution by them to the premium, but family members are not covered. It is of interest that all ambulatory and in-patient medical expenses are paid for by the insurance but meal costs in the hospital are excluded.

The second type of insurance, introduced in 1951 and revised in 1953, is called "labor medical insurance" (*laobao yiliao*); it covers workers and staff members in state-owned factories and enterprises.

The plan is financed by a percentage of income—estimated at 2 to 3 percent—of the factories and enterprises. Again there is comprehensive coverage and no "co-insurance" payment required from the worker. Dependents of the worker are covered by this plan but only to the extent of about 50 percent of their medical expenses. Since it is usual for both husband and wife to work, and often in the cities both work in state-owned enterprises, it is common to have comprehensive coverage without co-insurance for both parents and relatively good coverage for their children. Preventive care and other special services—such as contraception and abortion—are provided without charge.

The costs of medical care services are of course extremely low compared to costs in developed countries. The daily room charges at higher level hospitals are approximately one to two yuan. Chest surgery may cost about 30 yuan. Since the mean length of stay in hospitals is about two weeks, hospitalization for a serious illness may cost the patient some 50 yuan which may be more than a month's income for a peasant or worker. Some urban hospitals offer lower room rates to poor peasants and arrangements are made for deferred payment or even free care if there is no source for reimbursement.[17]

Overall, the number of hospital beds in China—urban and rural—increased rapidly from 1965 to 1980 (see Table 3 in chapter two). The ratio of beds, approximately 1,200,000 in the rural areas (one for roughly 700 people) and 800,000 in the cities (one for some 200 people), is lower than in the industrially developed countries (one for 100 people) but higher than the World Health Organization's estimate for the developing countries (one for 700 people).

The technical level of care, even in some of the higher-level hospitals, is still quite low; physicians from the U.S. have commented that hospitals are "20 to 30 years behind" those in the U.S. in many of their procedures and certainly in their amenities.[18] On the other hand, some technical procedures—such as open-heart surgery—that are performed in relatively few centers in China are performed at "world levels" and in certain techniques—such as microsurgery for replantation of severed limbs and treatment for severe burns—specific hospitals have made breakthroughs recognized and applauded in the most technologically developed countries.

As part of the intense effort to accelerate modernization and to import high technology from other countries it was announced in 1979 that a new medical center complex would be developed in Peking with a proposed completion date of 1984 or 1985. This new hospital was visualized as the eventual site of the facilities and faculty of the old Peking Union Medical College. Now known as the Capital Medical College of the Chinese Academy of Medical Sciences, it is the only medical college in China with an eight-year curriculum. An American committee was formed to assist in supplying the hospital with equipment and drugs from the United States; members of the committee included the president of the Squibb Corporation (a major pharmaceutical corporation), the former dean of the Harvard Medical School, and the director of the Massachusetts General Hospital.[19] This effort may have been slowed, or even postponed, as a result of the recent retrenchment in some modernization programs, but it is an indication of the direction in which many of the leaders of China's medical care system want to proceed.

Traditional Medicine

The policy toward traditional medicine might have moved in either direction during the Cultural Revolution. On the one hand, the emphasis on deprofessionalization, on decentralization, and on provision of medicine in the rural areas where Western-type technology was rare influenced the system toward increased use of traditional techniques. On the other hand, the attacks on the Four Olds (old ideas, old culture, old customs, and old habits) that was part of the period—and that led to destruction of some Buddhist temples and other ancient structures and relics—might have led to a campaign against "old" medical methods. The forces favoring traditional medicine, however, were clearly far stronger, and the late 1960s and early 1970s were a period of intense development and use of traditional Chinese medicine techniques. Doctors trained in Western medicine who had resisted learning or using traditional techniques were convinced to try them, and many found that the methods were indeed efficacious, particularly in conjunction with Western-type medicine.

Visitors in the early 1970s were repeatedly shown the results of this increased emphasis. There were numerous examples in almost every field of medicine.

Acupuncture. Acupuncture was used both for treatment of a wide variety of illnesses and for pain relief during surgery, a technique the Chinese called "acupuncture anesthesia."[20] In treatment, for example, visitors were brought to schools for deaf mutes and were shown children whose hearing and speech were said to have improved after acupuncture. Before and after data were, however, not available and questions about controlled studies were brushed aside. More convincing were demonstrations featuring patients with painful conditions such as arthritis who described the relief acupuncture had given them.

Both medical visitors and visitors who had never before been inside an operating room were shown multiple examples of surgical operations performed using acupuncture for pain relief. In contrast to the use of acupuncture in treatment, in which there was no way for the visitors to evaluate claims of efficacy, the evidence of visitors' own eyes showed patients undergoing major surgery with pain largely controlled by the insertion of a few needles. Doubters back home spoke of "trickery" or "hypnosis," but those, from many countries, who actually saw the surgery performed had no doubt that the needles were producing some form of pain relief.

The Chinese surgeons and acupuncturists explained that acupuncture was only used with selected patients, only with the patient's full cooperation, and only in selected types of surgery, such as that of the head, neck, and chest. During the surgery there was intense interaction between the medical personnel and the patient, including a full explanation of each step and often feeding the patient tea or fruit. Occasionally visitors were shown operations, such as the removal of an ovarian cyst, in which the pain relief was less than total.

Herbal Medicine. Even more common than the use of acupuncture was the use of medicinal herbs. Particularly in the rural areas, but also in urban health centers and even in urban hospitals, visitors were shown collections of chopped vegetable material such as roots, seeds, and bark—and at times ground animal material (such as horns) and minerals—stored in bins, drawers, and jars. When ready for use, the herbs were steeped in water, forming an "infusion," which was then consumed as a broth or a tea. Frequently prescriptions were very complex, with combinations of many different herbs in varying proportions.[21]

Flexible Splinting. The ancient technique of using flexible willow-wood splints was used for treatment of certain bone fractures. Articles on the technique had been published before the Cultural Revolution, for example, on its use in treating wrist fractures called Colles' fractures. In a series of 100 cases reported in the *Chinese Medical Journal* the author indicated that the results were better than in treatment of patients with the rigid casts used in the West.[22]

Other techniques. Among the other techniques shown to visitors were moxibustion, massage, and exercise. The diagnostic techniques of traditional medicine, including prolonged and detailed palpation of the pulse, were also widely used by its practitioners.

With the fall of the Gang of Four, criticism of the extensive use of traditional medicine during the Cultural Revolution period began to appear, with allegations that some of the reported successes of traditional medicine had been exaggerated. Nonetheless, traditional medicine continues to be actively used in a wide variety of circumstances. The *Chinese Medical Journal* reported in December 1980 that "more than 800 pharmaceutical factories throughout China now produce nearly 3000 types of traditional Chinese medical preparations."

Acupuncture is still employed for relief of pain during surgery, but apparently in patients who are more carefully selected for its use and therefore represent a smaller percentage of all surgical patients than was the practice earlier in the decade. Chinese publications have also now adopted the name acupuncture "analgesia" (pain relief) rather than acupuncture "anesthesia" (absence of sensation), a much more accurate representation of what is observed.[23]

Reports of the efficacy of acupuncture in treatment continue to appear, but still without the controls that Western physicians consider necessary to differentiate the specific effects of a treatment from natural improvements in the course of an illness or from "placebo" effects. Recent examples of reports of effective treatment include, for example, a report from the Acupuncture Research Institute of the

Academy of Traditional Chinese Medicine in Peking. In a study of 44 patients with angina pectoris and arrhythmia due to coronary heart disease treated with acupuncture, it was reported that 29 patients were "markedly improved," 13 "improved," and 2 "unchanged." The authors attempt to relate the traditional theory of channels running on the outside of the body connected with specific internal organs with modern evidence of nerve pathways in the body.[24]

Other research in China involves "humoral" theories of the action of acupuncture, such as the release of opiatelike substances in the blood or in the cerebrospinal fluid. Evidence for the humoral theories includes the ability to transfer the pain-relieving effects from an acupunctured animal to another animal by transfusion of blood or spinal fluid. The question is of course still unresolved, but it is widely believed—in China and in the West—that there are physiological as well as psychological factors responsible for the effects of acupuncture. International Acupuncture Training Courses, sponsored by the Ministry of Health under the auspices of the World Health Organization, are now conducted in Peking, Nanjing, and Shanghai; the course in April 1981 was attended by doctors from 18 countries, including the United States.

Research on traditional medicine is being increasingly encouraged. There are now five institutes affiliated with the newly strengthened Academy of Traditional Chinese Medicine. The work of one of the institutes, the Institute of Traditional Chinese Pharmacology in Peking, was described in *Beijing Review* in December 1980. The Institute employs 270 researchers with professional training in pharmacology, pathology, physiology, biochemistry, virology, clinical medicine, chemistry, or physics. Among the accomplishments of the Institute is the extraction of *ching hao su*, a new antimalarial drug. Its discovery is said to have been inspired by a medical work of the early fourth century. The drug is reported to have greater efficacy, more rapid effect, and lower toxicity than the widely used chloroquine. Among many other new drugs, a polysaccharide extract from a parasitic plant growing at the roots of some trees is said to have had proven anticancer effects in tests in 300 patients over a two-and-one-half-year follow-up period and the extract of the venom of a poisonous snake has been used as an anticlotting agent in patients with cerebral, retinal, and coronary thrombosis. In other work, a 3,000-year-old deep breathing exercise called *qigong* has been shown in controlled studies to reduce blood pressure in patients with hypertension; more than 10,000 people in Peking are reported to be performing *qigong* regularly.

In a combination of the traditional and the modern that raises other kinds of questions, it was recently announced that the Peking Traditional Chinese Medicine Hospital has stored in a computer "the diagnostic and treatment experiences of famous traditional Chinese doctors." A patient's symptoms can now be entered into the computer and a readout will give "the diagnosis, the prescription, and the doctor's advice." How this system will replace the long and detailed questioning and examination of the patient and the personal interaction around treatment between patient and doctor that appear to be essential components in the practice of traditional medicine is not, however, explained.[25]

In short, by every indication the Chinese plan to carry the attempt to study all forms of traditional medicine and their integration into "scientific medicine" into the new period of "modernization." Some problems with physician acceptance are said to remain but, unlike the pattern in most developing countries, the principle of "uniting" traditional medicine with modern medicine seems likely to be pursued.

Medical Personnel

During the Cultural Revolution, as part of the rethinking of all educational practices and in large measure because of the special attention given medical education in Mao's "June 26th Directive," no aspect of the educational system came in for more drastic "criticism, struggle, and transformation" than did medical education.

In 1968 the revolutionary committee of the Shanghai First Medical College, for example, analyzed medical education prior to 1966:

> ... Under its decayed system and time-worn methods (copied from capitalist and revisionist countries), were trained so-called "first-rate doctors" who were divorced from proletarian politics,

divorced from the workers, peasants, and soldiers, and divorced from practice—bourgeois intellectual aristocrats who rode over the working people and thought of nothing else than personal fame, wealth, and position. It ignored the five hundred million peasants and served only the cities. The curriculum required students to study as long as six or even eight years, but after graduation they were unable to treat independently even the most frequently encountered diseases. Leaving the big hospital, with its laboratories and modern equipment, they found themselves at their wits' end. In the course of six years, three fourths of the time was spent studying textbooks and reciting abstract theories. . .

Even during clinical study and internship they were still taught what had been copied from the capitalist and revisionist countries, such as separating medical science into numerous specialities, with the human body divided into as many airtight compartments. In treatment no consideration was given to what was best for the total patient. Under the domination of bourgeois intellectuals, students concentrated all their energy on the treatment of "rare diseases and difficult cases" and were oblivious of the commonly-seen diseases that most affect the working people. . .[26]

The China Medical College in Peking (in the buildings and with some of the surviving faculty of the old Peking Union Medical College), which in the early 1960s had instituted an eight-year medical curriculum oriented toward producing teachers and researchers, was particularly criticized. The editors of *China's Medicine* (which replaced the *Chinese Medical Journal* as the official organ of the Chinese Medical Association during the Cultural Revolution), in the introduction to an article "contributed by revolutionary students and workers at the college," alleged that the "reincarnation" of PUMC was "part of the criminal program . . . for restoring capitalism in the country." Among the points made in the article was that the leaders at the college

. . . invented the theory of "indirect service to the five hundred million peasants." Guided by this "theory," the college paid no attention to common ailments in the countryside but concentrated on "high standards." The students acquired skills that could be applied only in big urban hospitals.

As a result, none of the college's graduates over the years were assigned jobs in the countryside. When the revolutionary students rebelled and demanded that they be allowed to serve the peasants, the capitalist-roaders slandered them as "lacking in ideals." Some even said: "Do you think that we train you for eight years just to be country doctors?"

In the last analysis, "indirect service to the five hundred million peasants" meant "direct service to the bourgeoisie," and the theory of "cities before the countryside" meant refusal to serve the poor and lower middle peasants.

Of the new students enrolled in Peking between 1959 and 1962, only five percent came from worker or peasant families, while 30 percent came from families of top intellectuals. Children of bourgeois elements made up another five percent and children of landlords, rich peasants, counter-revolutionaries, bad elements and Rightists accounted for five percent of the total. The rest came from other sections of society.[27]

Starting in 1966, medical colleges admitted no new classes; students already in college were given accelerated programs of practical training and assigned to work in the countryside. Medical college faculty members, researchers in the institutes of the Academy of Medical Sciences, and other urban health workers spent periods in the rural areas performing manual labor and carrying out medical work such as training barefoot doctors, providing consultation and continuing education for medical workers, offering direct medical and preventive services, and mobilizing the peasants to play a major role in their own health care.

Intense struggle, including the public humiliation of teachers and administrators, was carried on in each medical college, and China's press and *China's Medicine* fanned the flames. Peking Radio Domestic Service in 1969 is quoted as saying: "It is imperative to completely change the educational system of old medical colleges and to make a thorough reevaluation of teaching content and methods." The Peking *People's Daily* published an article entitled "Medical Education Must Be Oriented Toward the Countryside and the Road of Integrating the

Western and the Chinese Schools of Medicine."[28] *China's Medicine* published articles such as "A New Approach to Medical Education," authored by the revolutionary committee of the "June 26th commune" of the Shandong Medical College, which cited Mao's statement that "there is no construction without destruction" and described a period of "great revolutionary criticism and repudiation" and of "mass debates on the question of whom medical education should serve and how the old system of medical education should be transformed."[29]

Groups of faculty members, students, and "workers, peasants, and soldiers" met to change admission policies and to shorten and restructure the curriculum. In an attempt to integrate traditional Chinese medicine into the curriculum, medical colleges brought in traditional practitioners as faculty members. A few colleges attempted to integrate their teaching with that of the college of traditional medicine in the same city, thus forming a college of "new medicine."

In 1969, on an "experimental basis," some medical colleges resumed admission of new students. The process of selection and the duration and content of the curriculum were markedly altered. Many of those admitted had not only not graduated from senior middle school but some had not even graduated from junior medical school. Each had worked in a commune or factory for at least two years and had been recommended as a candidate by the leadership of the commune or factory. No entrance examinations were given, a dramatic departure from the educational tradition of centuries. Selection criteria emphasized ideology, work record, and physical fitness. Academic ability was said to be a factor, but only to the extent of demonstrating that the student could handle the academic work in the medical school. Many of the new students had been health workers in their factories or communes. Of the 360 students enrolled in Peking Medical College's first post–Cultural Revolution class in December 1970, 80 percent had been barefoot doctors or other health workers and 55 percent were women.

Although each medical college had developed its own independent experimental curriculum, none of the schools we visited in 1970 and 1971 planned a curriculum beyond three years in duration. All had markedly reduced the curriculum time for preclinical sciences and had increased the time for political education and for training in traditional

Chinese medicine. All students were required to spend considerable time—in one school nine months of the three years—working and studying in the countryside together with their teachers.

When we asked how these colleges had managed to compress into three years material that had previously taken six years, we were told, "by eliminating the irrelevant and the redundant, by combining the theoretical with the practical, and by using the 'three-in-one' principle of teachers teach students, students teach teachers, and students teach students." The faculty of the Peking Medical College described in detail the elimination of the irrelevant and the redundant, and told us, for example, in how many different courses they had previously presented material on schistosomiasis. Overall, they said, "We used to require thirty-eight courses to teach a medical student; now we need only ten courses."

In 1971 we were told that there were no grades and no competition in medical colleges. There were indeed some examinations, but solely, we were informed, for the purpose of letting the students know what they had not completely understood and of letting the teachers know what subjects they were not teaching successfully. There was no reason for grades, it was said, because classes were small enough and faculty large enough for teachers to get to know the students well and to be aware of their progress. There was no reason for competition because the object was not for individuals to excel but rather to be good doctors.

By the time of our visit in 1972, based on one or two years experience with the new curriculum, leaders in the medical colleges we visited told us that the new students had been ill prepared to understand parts of the material and that the absence of examinations and grades led to inability of both students and faculty to evaluate the effectiveness of the teaching and learning. As a result some colleges, such as those in Xian and Peking, had instituted a six-month course, preceding the formal beginning of the medical curriculum, to provide additional background in the sciences and in a foreign language. At the Peking Medical College examinations were introduced at the end of each course and graded excellent, good, pass, or fail, or on a scale of 100 points. Our hosts still maintained that there was nonetheless little competition.

The pattern of admitting students from communes and factories, without entrance examination and, for many, without completion of senior middle school, continued through 1976. In our visits in 1977 and 1980, these classes of students were referred to as the "Worker-Peasant-Soldier" classes. They had been graduated after three to four years of medical education and most were now working in the countryside. In the late 1970s it was said that these students were viewed as incompletely prepared for medical practice and that upgrading courses were being developed to improve their knowledge and skills. Some faculty members with whom we discussed these graduates in 1980 compared them unfavorably to the "assistant doctors" who had been trained before the Cultural Revolution; they were said to be inadequate for fully independent medical practice.

Beginning in 1977 admission criteria and the curriculum for medical education were markedly changed. Entrance examinations are now given, only senior middle school graduates are eligible for them, and admission to medical college is entirely determined on the basis of the grades on the examination. The grade also determines to which medical college the student is admitted. Those with the highest grades are admitted to one of six medical colleges newly designated as "key schools": Peking Medical College, Peking Traditional Medical College, China Capital Medical University (the former Peking Medical College), Shanghai First Medical College, Sichuan Medical College (Chengdu), and Zhongshan (Dr. Sun Yat-sen) Medical College (Guangzhou). These colleges have higher priority for government funding and are to be developed as "model" medical institutions.[30]

The length of the medical curriculum in all medical colleges has been extended to five or six years, as it was before the Cultural Revolution. Time for theoretical and preclinical subjects has been expanded, with less emphasis on practical experience and political study and considerably less time spent in the countryside than in the early 1970s.

As discussed earlier in the chapter, one college—called in some descriptions the China Capital Medical University and in others the Capital Medical College of the Chinese Academy of Medical Sciences— was reactivated in 1979 as an eight-year medical school. The first 31 students, all from Peking, scored 400 or more out of 500 in the national admission examination in 1979. It is reported that, because of the large number of women in other medical colleges, "a deliberate effort was made to increase the number of men in the Capital Medical College student body, and preference was given to male candidates. If two applicants, one man and one woman, each scored 400 and all other variables were equal, the man was accepted."[31]

Since most of the work of the Chinese Academy of Medical Sciences is concerned with research rather than with service or teaching, it appears that the new college is in large part designed to train high-level medical researchers. Many will work after graduation in the research facilities directed by the Academy. The institutes and hospitals affiliated with the Chinese Academy of Medical Sciences and with the Chinese Academy of Traditional Medicine are listed in Appendix C.

In 1980 there were more than 100 medical colleges, listed in Appendix D, with more than 126,000 students and 2,700 postgraduates. With the establishment in 1978 of a medical college in Linzhi, a newly developed city east of Lhasa in Tibet, every one of China's provinces, municipalities, and autonomous regions has at least one medical college. Specialized faculties in medical colleges include those in the fields of medicine, pediatrics, public health, dentistry, traditional Chinese medicine, Chinese herbal medicine, and pharmacology.[32] Public health faculties in medical colleges admit 1,500 students annually. Overall, there was an increase of 36,000 doctors from 1978 to 1979 (a 10 percent increase) and of 52,000 from 1979 to 1980 (another 13 percent). China in 1980 had approximately one doctor for every 2,200 people (see Table 1 in chapter three and Appendix A). This is a much lower ratio than in the industrialized countries (which have one doctor for every 400 to 800 people) but much higher than the ratios for most countries at comparable levels of development.

China in 1980 also had 25 colleges for training doctors of traditional Chinese medicine as well as Uygur, Mongolian, and Tibetan medicine. These schools have a total enrollment of 20,000 and a small number of postgraduate students; the students are senior middle school graduates. The number of "Chinese doctors" increased by approximately 11,000 from 1978 to 1980 (a 4 percent increase), and there is now approximately one doctor of traditional Chinese medicine for every 3,700 people.

There are now some 400 "middle-level" or "secondary" medical schools in China, with ten specialty fields: medicine, gynecology and pediatrics, traditional Chinese medicine, public health, radiology, dentistry, nursing, midwifery, laboratory technology, and pharmacology. The students are mainly junior middle school graduates, but some are graduates of senior middle school; the duration of the curriculum is three years. Graduates work as assistant doctors, nurses, midwives, pharmacists, lab technicians, or other types of technical health workers.

It is of interest that though middle-level health workers are by far the largest single group of health workers, their numbers are increasing much less rapidly than those of either the "higher level" or "lower level" workers. The number of nurses, for example, increased by only 4 percent from 1978 to 1979, and 11 percent from 1979 to 1980, smaller increases than for doctors, even though there were in 1980 only slightly more nurses (466,000) than doctors (447,000) in China. At a recent meeting of nurses in Peking, the widow of Zhou Enlai "criticized the feudal attitude of looking down on nurses" and "called on the people working in various fields to show greater concern for the nurses in their work, study, and everyday life."[33] (In most industrialized countries there are considerably more nurses than doctors but many developing countries, which have greater difficulty recruiting women into nursing and are unlikely to use men in the role, have fewer nurses than doctors.) The number of assistant doctors rose at an even slower rate than that of nurses. The number of midwives—those with three years of training as contrasted with those trained for far shorter periods in the rural areas—rose by only 200 (0.3 percent) over the two years; since China's population rose by 2.6 percent over this period, there was actually a *decline* of the ratio of middle-level midwives to population. Among the middle-level health professionals, only pharmacists increased at the same high rate as did Western-type doctors. It is possible that in China one of the reasons for the relatively slow increase in number of most types of middle-level health personnel is their upgrading to the ranks of higher-level personnel.

The number of lower-level professional medical workers—not to be confused with the barefoot doctors and midwives working in the production brigades in the communes, who are not considered "professional" personnel—also increased significantly from 1978 to 1980, though not as rapidly as did the higher-level personnel. The number of lower-level "nursing workers" particularly increased, at a rate faster than that of middle-level nurses, suggesting a relative shift toward the use of what would be called "nurses' aides" or "practical nurses" in the United States, but the number of lower-level "laboratory workers" actually declined—simultaneously with a rapid rise in number of higher-level "laboratory doctors," and middle-level "laboratory technicians"— suggesting a shift toward much greater training for those staffing China's medical laboratories.

In short, training in the health professions shows many of the changes seen in the rest of China's educational system (see chapter seven) and suggests—over the two years at the end of the decade—a rapid shift, in everything but nursing, toward a much more technically trained, professionalized system. The changes are consistent with the recent developments in rural and urban medical care, and even with the current practice of traditional Chinese medicine discussed in this chapter.

4 | Put Prevention First!

As we have discussed, prevention has been of central importance in the provision of health services in China since the earliest days of the People's Republic and, in principle if not in social practice, for centuries before that. This chapter discusses programs and policies concerned largely with promotion of health and prevention of disease in communities. As in the last chapter we must emphasize the arbitrariness of this distinction. Occupational health services in China, for example, usually combine both personal medical care and efforts to prevent occupational disease. These services—and environmental health services, which are more clearly differentiated from personal health services—have been greatly expanded over the decade. Family planning services are similarly closely intertwined with personal health services. But in China such services are clearly a part of national policy and of a national effort unprecedented in any other country of the world. As the magnitude of China's population growth potential has become clearer in China over the decade, the program has become much more stringent and, apparently, increasingly effective.

The medical and health programs described in both the preceding chapter and this one, particularly their health promotion and disease prevention aspects, have clearly had a large impact on the health of China's people. But of even greater importance in the improvement of health, almost certainly, are the changes in literacy, in nutrition, in housing, and in social relationships that have occurred over the past thirty years. In this chapter, because it seems to fit best, we document the changes in the health of China's people, changes unprecedented among comparably poor countries in their breadth and rapidity. It must be noted, however, lest the inclusion of this section in this chapter be misconstrued, that we believe that the human services and educational policies discussed in the next three chapters, and other societal changes, have had as important an impact on the improvements in health as have the advances in the formally designated health services.

Environmental and Occupational Health

China made considerable progress in the 1950s and 1960s in solving its most serious environmental problems of that period, the ubiquitous agents and vectors of infectious disease. The work included extraordinary efforts to provide pure water and safe sewage disposal, particularly in the rural areas, and to eliminate flies, mosquitoes, and other "pests." The widespread spreading of nightsoil (human feces) as fertilizer required special attention; its use could not be avoided, but its hazards could be reduced by appropriate storage and treatment. Much of the preventive effort was conducted through mass movements and widespread popular participation; examples included the antischistosomiasis campaigns and the Great Patriotic Health Campaigns described in chapter two.

During the Cultural Revolution mass participation in pollution control appeared to continue and indeed expand. The consciousness of vast numbers of people, in both the countryside and the cities, was raised by their active involvement. For example, the Xinhua (New China) News Agency reported that in July 1968 the Shanghai Municipal Revolutionary Committee mobilized 90,000 people "from the industrial and agricultural fronts in Shanghai to form muck-dredging and muck-transporting teams, waging a vehement people's war to dredge muck from the Suzhou River. After 100 days of turbulent fighting, more than 403,600 tons of malodorous organic mire had been dug out."[1]

Public health officials in China in the late 1970s, however, emphasized a different aspect of the Cultural Revolution period. It is now said that the antiprofessionalism and the disorganization of that period led to inability to inspect and to maintain standards for industrial processes and that the result was a large increase in air and water pollution.

In the past few years there has been evidence that rapid modernization has led to increased problems with industrial pollution. In 1980 Li Chaobo, Director of the Environmental Protection Office of the State Council, reported that 10 million tons of soot are released annually by the industrial and household burning of fuel, while the sulfur dioxide released exceeds 15 million tons. Over 90 percent of industrial liquid waste is discharged, without treatment, into rivers, lakes, and seas directly or indirectly. Solid waste amounts to 200 million tons annually.[2]

Other reports indicate that China now has nearly 400,000 factories and mines; in 1979 an estimated 78.8 million tons of polluted water and 9,900 million cubic meters of waste gas were discharged from the factories daily, in addition to an annual 450 million tons of industrial residue. China's rivers, including the Changjiang (Yangtze), Huanghe (Yellow), and Huaihe, are polluted to varying degrees by industrial effluent. Air pollution in the cities is the result, among other factors, of what Chinese officials call the "irrational distribution of industries" and the use of coal as fuel by large numbers of people.[3] Reports have appeared of water pollution with organic chemicals, mercury, chromium, and other wastes and of air pollution with hydrogen fluoride, sulfur dioxide, and a number of other pollutants. The small number of motor vehicles—there are 3,000,000 bicycles in Peking but only 180,000 motor vehicles—helps to keep the air pollution problem from being worse than it already is, but the number of motor vehicles, particularly trucks and buses, is growing rapidly.

Efforts to control this pollution are being increased. The Standing Committee of the Fifth National People's Congress in 1979 approved China's first law on environmental protection. The law covers "the air, water, mineral resources, forests, grasslands, wild plants and animals, aquatic life, places of historical interest, scenic spots, hot springs, resorts and natural areas under special protection as well as inhabited parts of the country." The forms of pollution covered include "liquid and gases as waste, slag, dust, sewage, radioactive material and other harmful matter as well as pollution from noise, vibration and toxic odors."[4]

A number of methods are used to enforce the law. Organizations and individuals who have a good record in environmental protection are officially commended and rewarded. Products made from waste materials are wholly or partially exempt from taxation. Profit of factories making these products may be used for dealing with pollution and bettering the environment. Units that cause pollution may be subject to criticism, warnings, or fines, or may be closed down until corrective measures are taken. Leaders of units as well as individuals responsible for serious pollution that leads to loss of life or serious damage to agriculture, forests, animal husbandry, sideline occupations, or fishing may be held accountable both administratively and financially and may be subjected to criminal penalties. The law also stipulates that every citizen has the right to keep watch over the environment, to report violators of environmental protection regulations to the authorities, and to file charges against organizations or individuals in court.

A number of accomplishments have been reported. In Liaoning, China's most industrialized province, more than 300 antipollution projects were constructed in 1979 and 1980. In Shenyang, capital of the province, the metallurgical plant, for example, introduced equipment for converting sulfur dioxide into dilute sulfuric acid. The retrieved sulfuric acid is worth more than 9 million yuan annually and the plant is no longer a major polluter of the city's air.[5] The environmental protection bureau in Dalian (Dairen), the major port of the province, ordered a machinery plant to pay 100,000 yuan compensation to local farmers for allowing industrial effluent to pollute an irrigation reservoir and four wells; the plant was given six months to bring the pollution under control. The city government reportedly fined the Dalian oil transmission station 20,000 yuan for allowing seventeen tons of crude oil to leak into the sea on two occasions in 1980, and a 3,000 yuan fine was imposed on the Dalian metal processing plant, which discharged a large volume of acid water into a lotus pond in a park, killing the flowers and fish.[6]

Occupational health has also shown both marked improvements

and serious problems since 1949. The child labor and horrendous working conditions of pre–Liberation China have been ended and China's factories in general provide environments superior to those of factories in other developing countries. Nonetheless, considerable numbers of occupational injuries and illness occur, particularly in this period of rapid modernization. Western visitors have reported absence of basic elements of worker protection in many factories. Noise levels, for example, are often extremely high. In January 1980, a new regulation required that all new factories must keep the noise level to 85 decibels, and existing enterprises may not exceed 90 decibels; it was estimated that only 20 to 30 percent of China's factories were within the prescribed limits.

Research in occupational health is being actively pursued. A nationwide survey of occupational diseases was conducted in 1979–1980 and is expected to provide detailed information on health problems caused by silica, lead, benzene, and mercury. Research is also being conducted on engineering controls in workplaces to minimize worker exposure to occupational hazards. As an example, the *Chinese Medical Journal* in 1978 published an article describing a new device using a jet water spray to reduce the coal dust level in mines; the article was submitted by the Xuzhou Health and Anti-Epidemic Station, the Xuzhou Coal Mining Administration, the Chuantai Coal Mine, and the Xuzhou Medical College.[7] There are a number of other examples of such collaboration in environmental and occupational health research among public health, administrative, industrial, and educational institutions.

In sharp contrast to the still inadequate status of engineering controls, or even personal protective devices, for prevention of occupational disease and injury, personal health and medical care services in factories are widespread and intensive. Care for occupational illness and injury is combined with general medical care in the health stations and clinics of most large factories. Some of the largest factories also have a factory hospital with in-patient beds. Smaller factories often make special arrangements with neighborhood health stations and hospitals for care for their workers.

In the early part of the decade workers in many factories were trained in short courses to become "worker doctors," part-time health workers analogous to the barefoot doctors in the countryside and the Red Medical Workers in the cities. They provided general health education, preventive services, family planning education and contraceptives, specific occupational health promotion services, screening for illness (such as taking blood pressures), and treatment for minor illnesses and injuries. By the end of the decade, however, the worker doctors were being phased out and largely replaced by full-time professional health workers such as assistant doctors and nurses.

Extensive surveys are conducted to detect treatable illness and to engage workers in appropriate medical care. Examples include vaginal smears for the detection of uterine and cervical cancer and blood pressure screening for detection of hypertension. A blood pressure survey was conducted of 10,450 workers in the Capital Iron and Steel Complex in Peking in 1967–1971. The prevalence rate of hypertension (defined as diastolic pressure above 90mm Hg) was 12.1 percent among the male workers and 4.9 percent among the females. For those with diastolic pressure below 100mg Hg, "general advice and follow-up once every two months were given"; for those with diastolic pressures of 100 to 110mm Hg, antihypertensive drug treatment was initiated with monthly follow-up. Those with diastolic pressure above 110mm Hg and those with cardiovascular complications received drug therapy and were checked every two weeks. A five-to-seven-year follow-up published in the *Chinese Medical Journal* in 1979 indicated, for example, that "a large proportion of workers with diastolic pressures between 90 and 100mm Hg were found to have their blood pressures spontaneously changed to normal." Further studies are being conducted "to determine the precise level of diastolic pressure below which drug therapy is to be considered unnecessary on a community basis."[8]

In addition to this work in the factories, specialized occupational disease hospitals and research institutes are being developed. In Shanghai, for example, the municipal Institute of Labor and Occupational Health both conducts research on occupational diseases and operates an occupational disease hospital, and the Faculty of Public Health at the Shanghai First Medical College is involved in teaching and research in environmental and occupational health. In Peking, along with the work being done by the Faculty of Public Health at the Peking Medical College and other efforts at the municipal level, there is a Labor Protection Section of the Institute of Public Health (Hygiene) of the Chinese Academy of Medical Sciences (see Appendix C). The section has working groups on toxicology, dust, physiology, chemistry, and pharmacology.[9]

All medical expenses for workers in state enterprises—whether the illness or injury is work-related or not—are paid by the enterprise and, during treatment, salary is paid in full. If the worker recovers and returns to work, he or she is to be given suitable work by the management of the workplace. Large and "medium-sized" factories are also said to run sanatoriums and rest homes for workers while they cannot return to work.

China's trade unions, only recently reconstituted after their dissolution during the Cultural Revolution, also play a role in medical care for workers. It was recently alleged by the deputy director of the Labor Insurance Department of the All-China Federation of Trade Unions that the trade union sanatoriums and rest homes were closed during the "ten years of chaos" from 1966 to 1976 because the Gang of Four called them "hotbeds of revisionism." In 1980 the unions provided a total of 126 sanatoriums and rest homes, with 27,000 beds, that serve over 100,000 workers annually. Most of the sanatoriums care for workers with chronic illnesses such as arthritis, and digestive and respiratory disorders; others specialize in specific occupational diseases and hepatitis. The majority of the sanatoriums are located in scenic resorts with good climates.[10]

Despite all of these efforts, there remains a serious problem in China, with its current emphasis on rapid industrialization: the "contradiction" that many of those who plan the building of factories and many factory managers perceive between the high levels of production that are expected despite limited capital funds and the need for environmental and worker protection. In a society in which capital for construction of production facilities is extremely limited, the additional cost of providing for industrial pollution control and safety is apparently often resisted. In 1980, for example, a Chinese public health educator visiting the United States sought a "simple formula" with which to calculate the pattern of dispersion to safe levels of pollutants discharged into a flowing river. The object, he said, was to permit planners to locate new plants along the banks of a river and to use the river to dispose of the industrial wastes, without harming the environment and the people downstream. The U.S. experts who were asked this question advised that the river not be used as an industrial toilet and that alternative methods of detoxifying the wastes or of recycling them be found. The visitor from China responded that safer methods of disposal would cost the factory much more than release into the river—for some factories, he estimated, adding 50 percent to their capital cost and considerably increasing the operating costs—and that China simply could not, in the current state of its economy, afford this luxury. The river, he said, would simply have to do its part.

In short, the apparent contradictions between rapid industrialization—which many Chinese believe is indispensable to raise the standard of living of their people and for their defense—and protection of the environment and the worker seem to pose an increasing problem in China. The dilemma may be a real one for the individual factory or even an entire industry. But for the society as a whole there may be ways to avoid the dilemma, to provide sufficient jobs, to achieve adequate productivity, *and* to protect workers and environment. This would appear to require, however, a commitment to central planning and to selective development that may be incompatible with the amount of autonomy currently given to individual factories and industries.

Finally, one of the few harsh criticisms of China's health measures made by visitors early in the decade concerned the absence of any attempt to educate the population about the dangers of smoking cigarettes or to control their use. The response in China at the time was that lung cancer in China is relatively rare—even when, as discussed later in this chapter, considered as a percentage of all cancers—and that a pleasure denied to poor people before Liberation, that they now enjoyed, should not be denied without good evidence of harm. Arguments about the long latent period for lung cancer—the usual twenty years or more delay between start of smoking and the appearance of symptoms of cancer—did not appear to sway public health officials.

In July 1979 the Ministries of Public Health, Finance, Agriculture, and Light Industry issued a joint statement, approved by the State Council, warning about the "harmful effects" of smoking, advising the people to curtail smoking, and setting forth a series of measures to accomplish these goals.[11] This combination of ministries, Fox

Butterfield pointed out in the *New York Times,* is significant in that all but the Ministry of Public Health have a vested interest in cigarette production. China's tobacco output in 1978 was estimated at nearly a million tons compared with U.S. production of 910,000 tons. India, the world's third largest producer, is far behind with 430,000 tons. Cigarette production is a state monopoly, one of the more profitable ones, and cigarettes are heavily taxed.[12]

The campaign on smoking has been accompanied by the release of data on smoking and its effects. The State Planning Commission disclosed that retail sales of cigarettes in China were 4.6 million cases in 1965 and 11.5 million in 1977, an increase of nearly 150 percent. The Ministry of Public Health, in an interview, indicated that the incidence of lung cancer in Shanghai has increased sixfold in fifteen years and is increasing each year in Peking, Nanjing, and other cities.

Measures taken so far encompass major education efforts, production changes, and restriction of smoking in specific places. Education includes the introduction of curriculum material in schools; publicity on radio, television, and newspapers; articles in the publications of the Communist Youth League, trade unions, and other organizations; and the issuance in 1980 of two antismoking postage stamps. Production changes include limitation of the amount of nicotine in cigarettes (a measure of questionable value for the prevention of lung cancer but possibly otherwise useful), increased production of filtered cigarettes (which cost much more than ordinary ones), and provision of a type of chewing gum designed to help people stop smoking. Restrictions include prohibition of smoking in public places such as hospitals, theaters, movie houses, and kindergartens and "banning of smoking among all college students as a disciplinary measure."

These measures—while a dramatic change from the previous level of attention to the problem—still seem limited in a country that, in theory at least, has complete control over the industry and could presumably do more.

Family Planning

China's population policy has undergone numerous swings since the Communists took power in 1949. Due to increased and more equitable distribution of food, intensive sanitation, and other efforts to bring infectious disease under control, the combination of malnutrition and infection that kills so many people—particularly children—in poor countries was rapidly diminished. Mortality levels therefore fell sharply during the 1950s. At the same time an increase in marriages that had been postponed during the turmoil of the 1940s was followed by a sharp upsurge in births. There was consequently a significant rise in the rate of natural increase in the population of China by the mid-1950s. Although Mao and others within the government had dismissed birth control programs based on Malthusian fears as a program to "kill off the Chinese people without shedding blood," by 1956 birth control efforts were being promoted, though primarily in the urban areas. This effort was short-lived, since it was essentially terminated during the Great Leap Forward in 1958 (see Table 1).

A second birth control campaign was begun in 1962 but had almost no impact in the rural areas and, apart from major cities such as Shanghai, only slight impact on the urban birth rate. This campaign was disrupted in 1966 by the Cultural Revolution. In fact, it has been reported that during the late 1960s young people in some areas took advantage of the relaxation of administrative controls over marriage to marry and a significant increase in the number of births followed.

The third nationwide birth control campaign got underway in the early 1970s, just after medical and other institutions were reorganized following the upheaval of the Cultural Revolution. Late marriage was promoted (ages 24 to 26 for women, 26 to 29 for men); two or three children were considered the maximum, popularized through the slogan "two children per couple are enough, three are the limit and four is too many"; and lengthy spacing between children was encouraged. Workers at all levels of the political system and at all levels of the health care system were mobilized to educate the population about Chinese citizens' obligation to China to limit their number of children and the consequent need for family planning.

Contraceptives of various types were made available free of charge, were distributed by the barefoot doctors and midwives in the rural areas and by the Red Medical Workers in the cities, and were freely available in pharmacies. The most frequently used methods, based on limited data, were condoms, intrauterine devices, and oral contra-

Table 1
Population Growth*

Year	Total Population† (in millions)	Birth Rate** (per 1000)	Death Rate** (per 1000)	Natural Growth Rate** (per 1000)
1949	541.7	43	28	15
1953	588.0	37.0	14.0	23.0
1957	646.5	34.0	10.8	23.2
1978	958.1	18.3	6.3	12.0
1979	970.9	17.9	6.2	11.7
1980	982.6	n.a.	6.2	n.a.

†*At the end of the calendar year.*
**During the calendar year.*
Sources: Data for 1949–Population: China Encyclopedia Yearbook, 1980;
  Birth Rate: Leo A. Orleans, Every Fifth Child, *p. 49; Death Rate: "From 36 to 68,"* Beijing Review *24 (July 6, 1981): 4.*
  *Data for 1953 through 1979–*China Encyclopedia Yearbook, 1980.
  Data for 1980–Population: State Statistical Bureau, "Communiqué on Fulfillment of China's 1980 National Economic Plan," Beijing Review *24 (May 18, 1981): 20; Death Rate: "From 36 to 68,"* Beijing Review *24 (July 6, 1981): 4.*

ceptives. Diaphragms were used relatively rarely. Carl Djerassi estimated in 1973 that 15 million women in China used the pill, more women than in any other country in the world. Furthermore, the Chinese had introduced a low-dose combination pill at least five years earlier than its introduction in the United States.[13] Inexpensive methods were used, such as dipping a square of rice paper into the contraceptive steroid and ruling off 25 small squares, one to be torn off and taken on each of the first 25 days of the month. Sterilization was also made easily accessible for both sexes but, as in all countries, the number of tubal ligations far exceeded the number of vasectomies. Abortion during the first trimester was free and easily available, but women were urged not to use abortion as a primary contraceptive method and to attempt to limit its use to contraception failures.

These efforts led to a significant further fall in birth rate, from about 27 births per 1,000 population in 1973 (already, of course, markedly down from a reported high of 44 per 1,000 in 1963) to 18 per 1,000 in 1979. The overall death rate remained fairly constant during the decade, despite a relative aging of the population, at about 6 deaths annually per 1,000 population (compared to 14 per 1,000 in 1953). The natural population growth rate (the difference between birth rate and death rate) therefore fell from 21 per 1,000 in 1973 to 12 per 1,000 in 1979.

Despite this remarkable achievement, when the Second Session of the Fifth National People's Congress met in June 1979 it was clear that China's population growth would still be enormous. New population projections calculated within China—a resumption of work that was said to have been interrupted during the Cultural Revolution—had become available. Data published in the *People's Daily* in March 1980 indicated, for example, that if an average of three children per couple were maintained, China's population (not including that of Taiwan), which was estimated at 970 million at the start of 1980, would reach 1.4 billion by the year 2000 and 4.3 billion (the total *world* population in 1980) by 2080. Projections, shown in Figure 1, were also made for a variety of other fertility rates. They showed, to take an example from the other extreme, that if the number of children born were reduced dramatically to one child per couple by 1985 and maintained at that level thereafter, China's population would continue to grow for another 25 years and peak at just over 1 billion in 2004; it would then begin to fall, down to 370 million, approximately one third of China's current population, by 2080.[14]

The reason that population would continue to rise over the next 25 years even if children per couple were quickly and dramatically reduced—and that population would explode if fertility were not reduced—lies in the age structure of China's population. Although no formal nationwide census has been taken since 1957 and the census scheduled for 1981 has been postponed to 1982, samples of the national population in 1978 showed that 39 percent of the population was under the age of 15; the corresponding figure for developed countries is approximately 25 percent. This huge segment of the Chinese population has yet to reach childbearing age. Even more striking, in the years from 1954 to 1957 and 1962 to 1971 some 10 million more babies were born each year than in the intervening years. The children born during these high birth periods reach marriageable ages in peaks centering about 1980 and 1990. Thus a moderate lowering of children

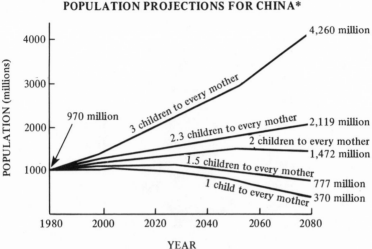

Figure 1
POPULATION PROJECTIONS FOR CHINA*

Source: Gerard Chen: Population Forecasts for China's Coming Century, Eastern Horizon 19 (4): 29–31, April 1980.

per couple would be vitiated by the number of new couples entering the childbearing years and the birth rate and population growth rate would continue to rise despite the efforts.

The problem is graphically demonstrated by population data for the Luwan District of Shanghai given to us during our visits in 1972 and 1980 and shown in Figure 2. In 1971 Luwan's population distribution showed a large number of people in the age range 8 to 20, i.e., those born from 1950 to 1962, and relatively small numbers of children aged 0 to 8, i.e., those born from 1963 through 1971, a period in which Shanghai maintained an intense birth control campaign. In 1979, the peak had shifted; people who had been aged 8 to 20 in 1971 had moved into the age range 16 to 28 and the effects were beginning to be seen in Shanghai's birth rate. Despite even more intense birth control efforts during the decade the birth rate had begun to rise in the late 1970s; only the extraordinary effort kept it from exploding.

Faced with these projections, the National People's Congress in

Figure 2
POPULATION DISTRIBUTION OF LUWAN DISTRICT, SHANGHAI*

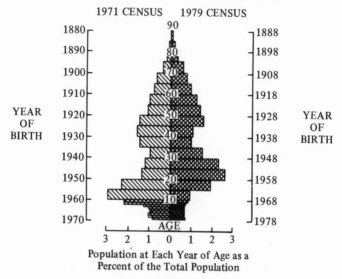

Population at Each Year of Age as a
Percent of the Total Population

*Source: Data supplied by Shanghai Bureau of Public Health.

June 1979 decided to launch a massive campaign to promote the one-child family. On June 18, 1979, Premier Hua Guofeng stated, "The State demands that each couple should ideally have only one child and not more than two. To produce a third child is to violate the State regulations."[15] Elaborate and varied incentives and disincentives have subsequently been developed to encourage couples of childbearing age to limit the number of their children to one. Couples who have had one child and then pledge that they will have no more are issued a "Planned Parenthood Glory Certificate" that entitles them to benefits in health care, housing, food allowances, and work assignments. Those who have two children will essentially break even; they will neither be rewarded nor lose benefits. Those who have three or more children after 1979, however, will lose benefits in a variety of ways. By late December 1979 the Chinese reported that over 4 million married couples of childbearing age with one child had pledged to have no more children and in January 1981 the number was said to be over 10 million. China's natural growth rate was reported as "less than 11 per 1,000" in 1980 and eighteen provinces and municipalities had reduced their growth rates to "less than 10 per 1,000."[16]

The rewards for agreeing to have only one child vary somewhat from city to city and from province to province. While material rewards have received the greatest amount of attention both in the Chinese and the Western press, in part because the use of material incentives for this purpose was such a departure from long-standing principles in China, the importance of nonmaterial incentives should not be minimized. In a society in which consensus, mass support of public campaigns, particularly health campaigns, neighborhood and workplace pressure to conform, and the esteem of one's neighbors are of great importance, active participation in an effort such as the one-child family campaign brings the couple praise and recognition both within their neighborhood and within their place of work.

According to the Committee for the Defense of Children, a Chinese governmental group concerned with issues involving children and families, the material incentives offered in Peking for those who have signed the "one-child pledge" include a monthly stipend of five yuan from the birth of the first child until that child turns fourteen, living space equal to that given to two-child families or priority in housing, six months of paid maternity leave (compared to the usual fifty-six days of paid maternity leave), totally free medical care for the child until age seven, and priority when the child seeks admission to school or applies for a job. In addition, an only child who lives in the city is exempted from future assignment to work in the rural areas. In Shunyi County, a rural county in the Peking Municipality, the economic rewards include five yuan per month from the birth of the first child until the child is ten years old, six months paid maternity leave for the pregnant woman, priority in nursery school and kindergarten admission and in housing and a bonus of 60 or 100 yuan at the time the couple applies for the single-child certificate. Some areas—but not all—have adopted provisional penalties, subject to modification based on experience, for those who have more than two children. In some areas, for example, workers who have more than two children may not receive promotions or increases in pay. It has also been reported from some areas that for those couples for whom the cost of delivering children is paid by the state or by the parent's workplace the cost of having any child beyond two children must be borne by the parents. In addition, a third child may not receive subsidized medical care and there is a limit on the number of children from a single family who can attend a university simultaneously.[17] Some of the penalties used in parts of China have recently been criticized; health workers have been urged not to resort to "coercion and commandism" but rather to focus on guidance and education.[18]

The most frequently used methods of birth control at the end of the decade were still oral contraceptives, intrauterine devices, and condoms. New methods, still experimental, introduced during the 1970s include a "male pill" (related to the cottonseed constituent gossypol), with which there are still some problems of toxicity, and a "vacation pill" (the synthetic steroid Anordrin) to meet needs of couples who work in separate cities and meet only on vacation.[19] Both male and female sterilization is encouraged, but most reports indicate that the number of tubal ligations performed during the 1970s continued to be much larger than the number of vasectomies. Oral contraceptives and condoms continue to be dispensed free of charge and without prescription at many pharmacies; packets of pills are available complete with instructions and men are encouraged to help themselves to condoms.[20]

A variety of techniques is used to educate the population about the importance of birth control. According to health workers in 1980 in the Fengsheng Neighborhood, where 88 percent of families with one child have applied for a one-child certificate and over 90 percent of the couples of childbearing age are using contraception, education methods include films, operas, seminars, and exhibits. In the health station of the Da Cheng Residents' Committee, part of the Fengsheng Neighborhood, health workers meet with couples in large meetings, in small meetings, and on a one-to-one basis to explain the importance of the one-child family. In the Da Cheng Residents' Committee there are 96 women of childbearing age who have one child; 91 of them have pledged not to have more children.

The one-child family is also stimulating efforts to persuade families that female infants should be as welcome as male infants. Job preference will be given to "only" children even if the child is a female, and to females who have no brothers. In the past a son had been expected to take over his father's job at the time of retirement; now a daughter may do so if she is qualified. Equal pay for women is being stressed, and husbands of "only" daughters are being encouraged to become part of their in-laws' households after marriage rather than following the traditional practice of a daughter-in-law moving in with her husband's family.[21]

The one-child family will also have an impact on the care of the elderly in China. Article 15 of the Marriage Law adopted on September 10, 1980, at the Third Session of the Fifth National People's Congress states, "Parents have the duty to rear and educate their children; children have the duty to support and assist their parents ... when children fail to perform the duty of supporting their parents, parents who have lost the ability to work or have difficulties in providing for themselves have the right to demand that their children pay for their support." These responsibilities will be far more difficult to carry out in an era of one-child families. If young people who are "only" children marry one another, they will be responsible for caring for two sets of parents; some parents may, therefore, have no children to care for them as they get older and society will need to take greater responsibility in their care.

Maternal and child health are being particularly promoted since the one-child family campaign. While the new Marriage Law stipulates that the legal age of marriage is twenty for women and twenty-two for men, late marriage and late childbirth have been advocated for a decade. Some leaders of the Women's Federation are, however, concerned about women giving birth to their first and only child when they are in their late twenties or early thirties. When parents are having only one child, they point out, that child must be healthy and they suggest that it might be preferable for childbirth to take place at an earlier age to maximize the health of the child and of the mother.

Rural health care is also being modified to support the one-child family. Midwives' training is being upgraded, and more deliveries are taking place in commune hospitals rather than at home or in brigade health stations. In the Yangzheng Commune in Shunyi County, for example, in the early 1970s 80 percent of the deliveries were in the home and only 20 percent in the hospital. By 1980 50 percent were taking place in the commune hospital.

Genetic counseling, a field that had been criticized and little practiced in China since Liberation, is currently being revived. Wu Min, a geneticist and professor in the Chinese Academy of Medical Sciences, has estimated that China now has over 10 million people with various forms of congenital defects. Chinese geneticists believe that since patients with congenital diseases who would have died as infants or children prior to Liberation are now surviving and marrying, the birth rate for congenitally deformed babies has increased. In addition, they believe that the "serious pollution of the environment," the practice of marriage between close relatives, and procreation by the mentally retarded cause an increase in the number of babies born with congenital disease.[22] In April 1979 the Genetic Research Institute and the Department of Gynecology and Obstetrics of the Number One Hospital attached to the Hunan Medical College began to offer genetic counseling to prospective parents on an out-patient basis. Using chromosome analysis geneticists advise parents when there is a known genetic defect in the child they are expecting and advise them in the decision whether to have an abortion or carry the baby to term.[23]

Concern with consanguineous marriage had apparently increased, at least in some quarters, by the end of the decade. The Institute of Genetics of the Chinese Academy of Sciences late in the 1970s conducted a survey of groups of minority nationality people in Gansu Province and found that marriage between close relatives constituted as much as 10 percent of all marriages. China's new marriage law prohibits marriage of "lineal blood relatives or collateral blood relatives (up to the third degree of relationship)." Geneticists in China are now advocating a "eugenics" law, such as the one enacted in Japan, that requires partners to exchanged medical certificates before marriage to ensure mutual knowledge of any hereditary disease. Some experts suggest that laws be passed "prohibiting the mentally retarded from procreating."[24] As the campaign for population limitation intensifies in China, it is being said that there should be "fewer babies but better babies."

In addition, the increasing availability of amniocentesis, with its ability to determine the sex of the fetus—combined with the traditional preference for male offspring—may lead to selective abortion of female fetuses. This, together with parents' decisions not to have a second child based in part on whether the first is a male, may produce gross distortions in male/female ratios similar to those produced by female infanticide.

There is one major exception to the intensive campaign for population limitation in China, which is largely directed at its ethnic Chinese population, also known as the Han people, who comprise 94 percent of China's billion people. The remaining 60 million are divided among 55 groups referred to in China as "national minorities." For them the population policy is quite different, as stated by the Xinhua News Agency in 1977: "In areas inhabited by the minority nationalists, many of whom were once dying out, the policy is to encourage population increase . . . However, guidance is available for those who wish to limit the number of their children." [25]

In summary, current policy in family planning for the Han population of China calls for "focus of family planning in the rural area," giving "favored treatment" to those who have only one child, strengthening of medical care for women and children, increased provision for the welfare of "old people without children," enhanced "research, production, and distribution of contraceptives," and the "raising of the technical level of the medical personnel involved in the work of birth control." [26] As to the future, a group of biological and social scientists at the third national symposium on population in Peking in February 1981 stated that the "optimum population" for a modernized China in the twenty-first century is 650 to 700 million. Their conclusion was said to be based on China's land area, its supply of natural resources, its rate of economic development, its environmental and ecological conditions, and on optional nutrition levels for its children. The symposium suggested that the target could be reached if over the next twenty years each couple bears only one child, holding China's population to 1.2 billion by the year 2000. Then it would become possible for couples to average two children, producing—because of the age structure of the population—a steady decline in the total to a stable 700 million by 2080. [27]

Health Statistics

The only health statistics provided to visitors early in the decade were those for specific, relatively small areas such as communes or cities. Aggregation of data beyond the local unit was apparently actively discouraged during the Cultural Revolution.

At times the quest for data became extremely frustrating for visitors. In 1971, for example, when we were told that there were no data on the number of preschool-age children in China we indicated our skepticism and our belief that such data had to be available in order to plan the production of sufficient doses of immunization materials. Our hosts responded that such production was based not on reports of the number of children but on the requests for materials from each individual unit. The requests for supplies were aggregated, not the data on population or illness, a concomitant of the decentralized planning and implementation of health services of the period. In other words, we were told that if planning is done locally there is no need for aggregation of the raw data on which planning is based.

Despite the paucity of data, those that were provided—such as infant mortality and other age-specific death rates for specific areas—were remarkably good for a country at China's state of development. Reports of these data simply whetted appetites for more.

Statistics on health in China at the end of the decade are still limited, but more complete data are rapidly becoming available. For some statistics, data are still provided only for specific cities or local areas; for others national data are now published regularly.

For infant mortality, it is reported that the rate in Peking City Proper, for example, has fallen from 118 deaths in the first year of life per 1,000 live births in 1949 to 10.4 per 1,000 in 1980, a figure comparable to those of the most industrially advanced cities of the world and substantially lower than infant mortality in New York City (14.6 per 1,000 for "white" and 18.2 per 1,000 for "nonwhite" babies). But the 1980 rate for the entire Peking Municipality was reported as 14.8 per 1,000, suggesting that the rate in its rural area is close to 20 per 1,000.[28]

Infant mortality rates for Shanghai City Proper, shown in Figure 3, demonstrate a similar fall. It is important to note that the neonatal mortality rate—the death in the first 28 days of life per 1,000 live births—is now about three-fourths the infant mortality rate. This again is the pattern seen in industrialized countries, where most infant deaths occur in the first month of life, often due to congenital defects, in contrast to the pattern in developing countries where infant deaths, largely due to malnutrition and infection, continue during the entire first year.

Figure 3
INFANT DEATH RATES FOR SHANGHAI CITY PROPER*

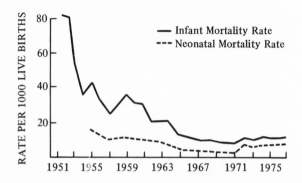

Source: Shanghai Bureau of Public Health, 1980.

Precise data on infant mortality rates have not yet been made officially available for all of China, but it was recently officially reported that infant mortality in China's cities had fallen from 120 per 1,000 in 1949 to 12 per 1,000 and had fallen in the countryside from about 200 per 1,000 in 1949 to 20 to 30 per 1,000.[29] These data, if confirmed by more precise figures, are considerably lower than those in other countries at China's level of economic development.

A more pessimistic estimate of China's infant mortality rate, published by both the Washington-based Population Reference Bureau and the World Bank (shown in Table 2), nonetheless also suggests that China is doing relatively well compared to other countries at its stage of industrial development. These agencies estimate China's infant mortality rate as 56 per 1,000 and its gross national product per capita as $260. With the exception of Sri Lanka, countries with comparable gross national products per capita have infant mortality rates far higher than those of China.

Overall death rates (technically called "crude death rates") are poor measures of health because they are generally more dependent on the age distribution of the country's population (countries with

Country	GNP per Capita (US dollars, 1979)	Crude Birth Rate (per 1,000 population, 1979)	Crude Death Rate (per 1,000 population, 1979)
India	190	34	14
Malawi	200	51	19
Rwanda	200	50	19
Sri Lanka	230	28	7
Benin	250	49	19
Mozambique	250	45	18
Sierra Leone	250	46	19
China	260	18	6
Haiti	260	41	14
Pakistan	260	44	14
Tanzania	260	46	15
Zaire	260	46	18
Niger	270	52	22
Guinea	280	46	20
USSR	4,110	18	9
United Kingdom	6,320	12	12
Japan	8,810	15	7
United States	10,630	17	9
Sweden	11,930	12	12

Sources: The data in Table 2 are largely drawn from the World Bank's World Development Report 1981. *Those marked with † are taken from the 1980 World's Children Data Sheet of the Population Reference Bureau; some of the latter may be from several years ago and are therefore not directly comparable with China's current data. Where separate figures for males and females were given in the sources, the male figures (usually more favorable) were used. The estimate of $260 for China's per capita GNP used by the World Bank is based on official figures released by China for 1979. Other estimates of China's GNP are higher. For example, the U.S. government estimate (from the National Foreign Assessment Center, Central Intelligence Agency) for 1978 was $444 billion (A. Doak Barnett,* China's Economy in Global Perspective, *Washington, D.C.: Brookings*

LE 2
Comparisons*

Infant Mortality Rate (per 1,000 live births, 1978)	Life Expectancy at Birth (years, 1979)	Daily Calorie Supply Per Capita (% of requirement, 1977)	Children Enrolled in Primary School (% of age group, 1978)	Adult Literacy Rate (percent, 1976)
125	52	91	79	36
142†	47	90	59	25
127†	47	98	64	24†
49	66	96	94	85
149†	47	98	60	12†
148†	47	81	53†	15†
136†	47	93	37	10†
56	64	104	93	66
130†	53	93	58	29†
142†	52	99	51	24
125†	52	89	70	66
171†	47	104	90	15
200†	43	91	23	8
220†	44	84	34	20
36†	73	135	97	100
14	73	132	106	99
9	76	126	98	99
14	74	135	98	99
8	76	120	99	99

Inst., 1981). China's per capita GNP based on this estimate was approximately $450. Use of the higher figure does not, however, change the conclusion that the health of China's people is substantially better than that of people of countries with comparable GNP per capita. For infant mortality rates and life expectancy, for example, countries in the $450 per capita income range include Ghana ($400), 115 deaths per 1000 live births and 49 years; Yemen Arab Republic ($420), 160 and 42; Senegal ($430), 160 and 43; Angola ($440), 192 and 42; Zimbabwe ($470), 129 and 55; Egypt ($480), 85 and 57; People's Democratic Republic of Yemen ($480), 170 and 45; Liberia ($500), 148 and 54; and Zambia ($500), 144 and 49, compared to the estimate for China of 56 and 64.

higher proportions of older people will generally have higher crude death rates) than on its death rates at each age. China's rate is reported to have fallen from 28 per 1,000 population in 1949 to 6.2 per 1,000 in 1980, a much greater fall than can be accounted for by changes in age distribution alone.[30] China's current crude death rate, as shown in Table 2, appears to be lower than those of countries of comparable wealth and age structure.

Life expectancy at birth is a better comparative measure than crude death rate because its method of calculation makes it independent of the age distribution of the population. Life expectancy at birth in China before Liberation is of course unknown, but it has been estimated at about 35 years; recent studies in China suggest that in 1981 it was 69.6 years for women and 67.0 years for men.[31] The World Bank's estimate (for 1979) is somewhat lower, but still much higher than their estimates for all countries of comparable economic development except Sri Lanka.

In addition, estimates of life expectancy at birth are available for specific cities in China. Life expectancy at birth for urban Peking, for example, has risen from 54 years in 1950 to 74 years in 1975 for males and from 50 years (1950) to 73 years (1975) for females.[32] For the entire Peking Municipality, including its rural areas, the estimate in 1980 was 70 years for males and 72 for females,[33] suggesting—as did the infant mortality data—that life expectancies in rural areas, even in the area surrounding Peking, are still significantly less than in urban areas.

Causes of death in China have of course changed markedly. In Shanghai, as shown in Figure 4, the leading causes of death in order of highest frequency are now cancer, stroke, and heart disease; in the United States the order is different—heart disease, cancer, and stroke— but the three leading causes are the same. The "main causes of death" in Peking in 1978 were reported to be "diseases of the heart and blood vessels and cancer."[34] While this is almost certainly not true for all of China, the trend is rapidly heading in that direction, representing a remarkable change from the infectious diseases, combined with malnutrition, that produced the bulk of deaths 30 years ago.

Cancers of the gastrointestinal system—particularly those of the esophagus and stomach—and of the nasopharynx occur in China at rates that appear to exceed those in other countries. For some cancers the

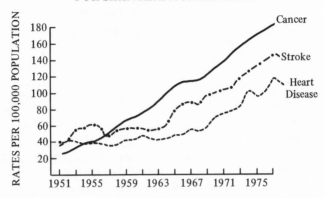

Figure 4
CAUSE–SPECIFIC MORTALITY RATES
FOR SHANGHAI MUNICIPALITY

Source: Shanghai Bureau of Public Health, 1980.

areas of high incidence are extremely concentrated. This is believed to be due to cancer production by environmental factors, and the very low geographic mobility in China, so that the end results of the factors are seen in the same locality many years later.

(In the United States, lung cancer is the leading cause of cancer death among men; it caused some 34 percent of all male cancer deaths in 1981. Among women, cancer of the breast (19 percent of all 1981 female cancer deaths) and of the lung (15 percent) are the leading causes of cancer deaths; lung cancer will by 1985 replace breast cancer as the most common cause in women.)

Community control programs for cancer, hypertension, and cardiovascular and cerebral vascular disease have been developed. Linxian (Lin County) of Henan Province has by far the highest reported esophageal cancer rates in the world, with age-adjusted mortality rates of 255 per 100,000 for males and 161 per 100,000 for females; approximately one out of every four deaths in the county is due to cancer of the esophagus. Intense efforts to find the cause of the cancer and preventive efforts—related to storage of grain to prevent fungus growth—have been initiated. In addition there is an extensive community effort to detect the cancer early so that it can be removed before it has spread locally or metastasized. Detection methods include education of the population to report specific symptoms as early as possible and a widespread screening program using a balloon with an abrasive surface that the patient swallows deflated and is then partially inflated so that cancer cells will adhere to it as it is withdrawn. The technique is less uncomfortable than it sounds, is widely accepted (in part because the barefoot doctors have an important role in its use), and has been highly successful in early detection.[35]

Community control measures for hypertension, stroke, and coronary heart disease have been developed in the Shijingshan People's Commune of the Shijingshan District, Peking Municipality. During the five-year period ending December 31, 1979, blood pressure screening was carried out twice in everyone over the age of 15. The prevalence of hypertension found, using World Health Organization criteria (systolic pressure 160mm Hg and/or distolic blood pressure 95mm Hg), was 5.5 percent. If "borderline" hypertension (pressure between 140/90 and 160/95) is included, the prevalence was 7.4 percent. At ages older than 25, women had slightly higher prevalence rates than did men. The prevalence of hypertension among peasants in the commune was significantly lower than the rates found among workers in an iron and steel plant located nearby (see data earlier in this chapter) and the rate found in a survey of the Peking urban population. The commune members not only showed a lower rate but a ten-year delay in onset; the marked rise in pressure in the peasants began at age 45; the marked rise in the urban and worker population at age 35.

Hypertension in the commune was treated by several methods. "Good results" (defined in the report) were obtained in 39 percent of the patients, "fair results" in 26 percent and "poor results" in 35 percent. The investigators call for "further efforts" to deal with those with poor results, but overall this effort and others among the commune members have brought a 23 percent reduction in mortality rates from stroke (which had been the leading cause of death in this commune) and a 13 percent reduction in mortality rate for all cardiovascular disease. It is of interest that after the five-year period the overall mortality rate in the commune changed very little; the mortality rates for cancer and for respiratory disease showed a significant rise. Some of these latter changes are almost certainly due to a rising age structure in the commune, as people on the average live to older and older ages, but the control measures appeared nonetheless to have an important impact.[36]

Despite the fall in infant mortality, the increase in life expectancy, and the rise in the importance of degenerative diseases, infectious disease remains a serious problem in China (see Appendix E). In 1978 there were 10,000 reported cases of poliomyelitis, 20,000 cases of diphtheria, 600,000 cases of whooping cough, and 1,100,000 cases of measles, all preventable illnesses. Although the incidence of these illnesses fell in 1979 and 1980—reported new cases of diphtheria, whooping cough, and measles fell by 50 percent and polio by almost as much—the data suggest that immunization campaigns are not yet as complete or effective as China would like. Other infectious diseases have higher incidence, and some are increasing; from 1978 to 1980 the number of reported cases of malaria rose from 3.1 million to 3.3 million (although there was a dip in 1979); cases of "dysentery" rose from 2.6 million to 2.9 million; and cases of infectious hepatitis from 411,000 to 475,000. Although their incidence is reported as decreasing, tuberculosis and trachoma are also said to remain problems. On the other hand, China reports little or no incidence of venereal disease, a serious infectious disease problem in both developing and technologically developed countries.

Nutritional deficiency diseases, once a large part of China's misery, are reported to be much reduced. The incidence of pellagra (a Vitamin B deficiency disease) and of rickets (Vitamin D deficiency) is markedly lower. Some 130 million people have specifically been provided preventive measures against iodine deficiencies that might in the past have led to goiter and even to severe consequences of thyroid hormone deficiency.[37]

The preceding data, while generally called "health statistics," are really morbidity and mortality statistics. Data on positive health, in every society, are much harder to obtain. One measure of health is the growth and development of children. Improvements in growth and development almost certainly owe more, of course, to changes in nutrition and to other aspects of child care than to specific health care services. Whatever the reasons, however, it is clear that growth and development of children in China improved markedly over the past 30 years.[38] The height and weight of Chinese children found in surveys are now comparable to, or higher than, those of children of Chinese parents in considerably wealthier societies.

Surveys—said to be the "most comprehensive ever carried out in China"—were conducted in 1979 by the health departments in nine major cities and in a nationwide study of 28 million preschool children in urban and rural areas. Barefoot doctors played an important role in the surveys; in Inner Mongolia, for example, medical teams visited the settlements of herdspeople and "checked the development, diet, and health" of 16,000 children under the age of seven. For China as a whole, the children were found on the average to be two centimeters (about one inch) taller and one kilogram (about two pounds) heavier than were children 30 years earlier. It is of special interest that development in girls, who had lagged behind boys, and of children in southern China, who had lagged behind those in northern China, has shown the relatively greater improvement. In Nanjing, for example, nine-year-old boys are on the average 4.6 centimeters taller and 3.1 kilograms heavier than nine-year-olds 30 years ago; girls of the same age average 5.4 centimeters taller and 2.8 kilograms heavier.[39]

In short, although a number of statistics show startling improvements in the health of the Chinese people over the past 30 years, there are still, especially in rural areas, high rates of infectious disease, including some that are clearly preventable. Even more disturbing, the incidence of some communicable illnesses, such as infectious hepatitis, appears to be increasing. The health status of China's population appears to be far better than that of 30 years ago and of people in comparably poor countries, but further improvement—especially for rural people—appears to be needed. In urban areas—and increasingly in rural areas—the leading causes of death and disability are the degenerative diseases of older age. Prevention of these illnesses, and of the disability associated with them, requires different types of efforts, such as prevention of cigarette smoking, reduction in industrial pollution, avoidance of obesity, and early detection and treatment of hypertension and of treatable cancers. China is beginning to make notable efforts in these fields as well.

III | Human Services

5 | The Individual, the Group, the Community: Problems of Daily Life

In attempting to organize their cities, Chinese leaders have been guided by two central principles: the establishment of a complex and extensive bureaucracy, as was common in traditional China, and the involvement of people in their own governance. Urban organization in China over the past thirty years has been, in large part, an effort to balance and blend popular participation and direction from above. The alternating emphases on bureaucratic organization or on mass participation closely reflect political events and ideology in China. The emphasis on antielitism and popular participation during the late 1960s and early 1970s was reflected in the cities in increased power at the local level; the current emphasis on rapid modernization, efficient management and increased production is reflected in greater centralization and professionalization of services and resumption of administrative control by higher levels of government. Both mass participation and close control over neighborhood life, however, remain important aspects of urban organization.

History of Urban Organization

The history of China's cities, like that of its medicine, stretches back nearly four thousand years. Many of today's important metropolitan and industrial centers were old county capitals and have survived successive dynasties, preserving a continuity from ancient times until today. Urban dwellers in traditional China were ruled indirectly through guilds, occupational groups, family clubs, and clans. When Chiang Kai-shek's Kuomintang assumed power in the 1920s, it took over existing forms of urban organization and extended city government further downward by dividing the cities into districts. Below the district level the only subdivisions were the police stations that were established in various sections of the city and were responsible for supervising the urban population.

In the first decade after they assumed power in 1949, the Chinese Communists faced severe problems in their attempt to govern the cities. During the Civil War that followed the Japanese occupation, inflation had become rampant, food was scarce, and services had broken down. Therefore, the new government needed to reconstruct services in the cities, maintain order, cope with increasing rural-urban migration, and mobilize the population to participate in the building of a socialist state.

When the government was finally able to establish order in the cities, local police stations began to take on civil responsibilities and mass organizations led by local party members or activists were formed to meet specific needs in health or sanitation. These efforts, however, were fragmentary, since leadership in any one neighborhood was not unified.

In December 1954, a series of governmental directives was issued by the standing committee of the National People's Congress delineating the future administrative framework of China's cities. Subdistrict offices would be established as local branches of the city government in all the major cities of China. They were mandatory in cities with over 100,000 population, optional in cities between 50,000 and 100,000 population, and not expected in cities of fewer than 50,000. Officials of the subdistrict were selected by the district city government, not by the residents.[1] Below the subdistrict, residents' committees were organized for the purpose of mediating disputes, organizing literacy classes and sanitation work, and dealing with welfare problems. The residents' committees were basically a device for organizing the unorganized, a group largely composed of unemployed women and the elderly. They were run by members of the masses themselves and, from the start, women played an important role in the workings of the residents' committee, often gaining power at that level when they had little at higher levels.

By 1957 rural-urban migration had increased significantly and large numbers of unemployed dependents of urban workers had crowded into the cities. Official data, based in part on the 1953 census and on population registration, indicate that the urban population rose at a rate of 7 percent per year from 1949 to 1957, compared to a mean annual rural increase of 1.4 percent. The urban population rose from 58,000,000 in 1949 to 99,000,000 in 1957.[2] To meet the needs of this new urban population, the Chinese government tentatively and experimentally established urban communes, a counterpart to the communes being established in the rural areas. This was the time of the Great Leap Forward, a time of hope that a truly integrated way of life—one that would combine work and leisure, physical and intellectual endeavors—might be at hand. But contradictions existed in the structure of the urban communes with regard to administration, production, and living, and ultimately the urban commune movement failed. Efforts toward developing a model of an integrated way of life based around work were largely discontinued; China's urban neighborhoods today are predominantly organized around residential areas rather than around production.[3]

At the end of the commune experiment, the Chinese government was still faced with the problems it had faced in the early 1950s: the problem of creating sufficient urban employment to match the rising urban population and the problem of creating a sense of community that would reduce the feelings of anomie and alienation characteristic of cities in both the West and the East. By the early 1960s the urban population had reached 130 million, approximately 20 percent of China's people. In response, migration from the countryside to the cities was sharply limited and a major rustification effort began. Between early 1962 and early 1964, 292,000 secondary-school graduates were resettled in the countryside; during 1964, more than 400,000 primary- and secondary-school graduates were resettled; and in the first eight months of 1965, 250,000 more graduates were sent out of the cities.[4] The target populations for this rustification movement, which was originally launched in 1957, were educated youths who had not yet been assigned jobs in the cities, young people who were neither attending school nor working steadily, and cadres whose skills were not needed in the cities but were needed in the countryside. There were several reasons behind the rustification effort: the transfer of resources from urban areas to rural areas; the education of urban youth about the reality of life in the countryside; and, of no small importance, the diminishing of pressure on overstrained urban services and job resources. Urban youths were, however, frequently reluctant to leave the relatively comfortable urban life surrounded by family and friends for an unknown, far more primitive life in the countryside.

During the Cultural Revolution, despite its emphasis on the rural areas, the Chinese continued to grapple with the issues of urban organization. With the onset of the Cultural Revolution, residents began to protest what they felt to be abuses on the part of the local neighborhood cadres. It was felt that cadres had become an entrenched group that had subtle advantages over the rest of the population, that they had lost contact with the people, and that they along with other Communist Party members and professionals were becoming a new elite.

One of the primary goals within the urban neighborhoods during the Cultural Revolution was to democratize the leadership and assure greater participation on the part of the masses. During the urban commune period, leaders of the residents' committees had been elected by the people, but members of the subdistrict committees were usually appointed by the district-level authorities. Even at the residents' committee level the candidates were often suggested by Party members, and in this way cadres and Party members exercised informal control. The consolidation of this informal control by the local elite during the urban commune movement was severely criticized during the Cultural Revolution. Residents also protested the scarcity of employment in the local neighborhoods and the massive mobilization of students to work in the countryside and in the border areas.

As other segments of Chinese society suffered from excesses and abuses during the Cultural Revolution so did the urban neighborhoods. Red Guards, students from the local schools, rampaged through courtyards searching out and destroying the Four Olds (old ideas, old culture, old customs, and old habits). According to one Red Guard:

Usually we began at one end of a street and worked our way to the other end. Using the police records as guides, we hung signs on the gates of every house that held a Black element ... We would then go back and search each house individually for old things ... In practice, we confiscated things like vases and furniture decorated in the traditional way. If they had revolutionary decorations, like pictures of Mao Tse-tung [Mao Zedong] or PLA [People's Liberation Army] men, we left them alone. Statues and religious articles were either confiscated or smashed.[5]

Shanghai's first revolutionary committee was established in Kuling Road in the densely populated Huangpu District in May 1967. The twenty-two-member committee, representing a constituency of 46,000 people, was composed of sixteen representatives of various local mass organizations, three representatives of the district organizations of government workers, and three representatives of local revolutionary organizations.[6] During the early period of selecting revolutionary committees, debates and wall posters discussing the merits and deficiencies of the candidates were very much part of the process. However, even when residents were in a position to participate alongside cadres, they still felt grossly inadequate. To encourage greater responsiveness to the needs of their constituents, members of the revolutionary committees were encouraged to go door-to-door to listen to the opinions and views of the people.

By 1968 the organization of neighborhood revolutionary committees was widespread. In Peking, for example, the Fengsheng Neighborhood is illustrative of both the changes in urban organization which took place as a result of the Cultural Revolution and the changes which have taken place in the four years since the death of Mao Zedong, the overthrow of the Gang of Four, the rapid drive toward modernization, and the repudiation of the Cultural Revolution.

Peking City Proper is divided into ten districts. The Fengsheng Neighborhood, located in the West District, covers 1.5 square kilometers and contains two main streets and 132 lanes. A lane (*hutong*) is a narrow street, usually with high gray walls on both sides; every few yards a door opens into a courtyard in which the people live. In 1972 the Fengsheng Neighborhood had a population of 53,000.

The Fengsheng Neighborhood had a leading body of twenty-seven members who were elected in March 1968. Seven members were full-time cadres; the other twenty were part-time members of the committee. Ten of the twenty-seven members were government cadres selected by the district level and sent to the Fengsheng Neighborhood to work. In addition to the ten government cadres on the committee there were two members from the People's Liberation Army and fifteen representatives of the mass who were selected by the units in which they lived or worked.

In 1972 the neighborhood committee was responsible for administering six factories which employed fifteen hundred workers; the nurseries, kindergartens and primary schools in the area; and one service department including eight service stations such as a watch repair shop, a clothing repair shop, and a shop to repair electrical appliances. The committee also administered the neighborhood hospital, the lane health stations, the housing management department, and one production group, a home industry for women who wished to work in their homes. In addition, the neighborhood was divided into twenty-five residents' committees ranging in size from four hundred families in the smallest residents' committees to eight hundred families in the largest.

The Fengsheng Neighborhood Hospital had one representative on the neighborhood committee, and the service department had one representative. One "housewife" was chosen for every two or three residents' committees. While the neighborhood was governed by representatives sent down from district-level committees and by representatives indirectly elected by the people living in the neighborhood but approved by committees at the district level and by the Party, it was extremely difficult to assess the relative strength of these two groups on the neighborhood committees.

Although some of the services provided by the neighborhood were subsidized by the district, during the late 1960s and 1970s the neighborhood committee had at least partial responsibility for income and expenditures relating to neighborhood services. For example, the lane health workers, known then as Red Medical Workers, were paid a modest stipend, which came partly from the small payments made by patients visiting the lane health station and partly from neighborhood-run industry. Nurseries and kindergartens run by the neighborhood committees were supported mainly by fees the parents paid and, if necessary, by supplementary aid from the funds of the neighborhood committee. While the neighborhood did not have full financial control over its services, it did have substantial financial control and therefore some legitimate authority over the form and substance of the services themselves. During this period the urban neighborhoods in China in fact gained some measure of community control over basic services and policies.

The residents' committees continued to be responsible for the elderly, students, and the few women of working age who remained at home. Working men and women remained under the aegis of their groups in their places of work. The leaders of the residents' committees were usually middle-aged women, who were no longer part of the labor force. They were not generally Party members but had been active in the community and related well to their neighbors. These local leaders were responsible for organizing study sessions, organizing sanitation work, and informal mediation of disputes between children, families, and marital partners.

In addition to these tasks, residents' committee members were expected to check on the presence of illegal residents in their lanes, protect the neighborhood from thefts, and generally keep the peace. The social control aspects of residents' committee work are vividly described by a woman who was a member of a residents' committee in Shanghai during the mid- and late-1960s and who has since moved to Hong Kong:

It was no secret that the people didn't always welcome our presence ... Most residents felt that the committee spent more time poking its nose into personal business and prying into people's lives than in acting on behalf of the residents. One of my neighbors asked me bluntly before I took the job, "Do you really want to do this? Your relations with your friends won't be the same anymore. They'll never speak their minds when you're around. They'll always think of you as someone who is going to cause them trouble. You know how people feel about the residents' committee; it's like a little policeman always checking up on us."[7]

The Current Scene

The changes in Chinese policy since the death of Mao have been reflected in urban organization as they have been reflected in other aspects of the society. In 1979 neighborhood revolutionary committees were abolished throughout China and subdistrict offices were reestablished in the neighborhoods, a reversion to the same organizational structure used prior to the Cultural Revolution. Today the lowest level of state power in the cities is no longer the neighborhood but is rather the district level; the administration of the neighborhood is through an office of the district level located in the neighborhood, called a subdistrict office. The major consequence of the reorganization has been the return of the administration and control of professional and quasi-professional services to specialized professional auspices at the district level as they were prior to the Cultural Revolution rather than their remaining under the "unified" leadership at the neighborhood level as they had been since the onset of the Cultural Revolution.

There is considerable confusion around the appropriate terminology to use in English to designate the various levels of urban organization. During the Cultural Revolution the area governed by the lowest level of state power (on the order of 50,000 people) was the *jiedao* (literally, "street"), the name of whose governing body was sometimes translated as "neighborhood committee," sometimes as "street committee." Since the abolition of the revolutionary committees at this level, the subdivisions of the urban districts are governed by what *Beijing Review* calls "Neighborhood Agencies," which they attempt to clarify by adding the designation "District Government Arms."[8] The next lower level, formerly called "residents' committees" (governing approximately 2,000 people), is now called "neighborhood committees." The lowest level (100-200 people) continues to be termed "group." Because of the confusion engendered by the dual use of the word "neighborhood," we limit our use of the term to designate the geographic areas (approximately 50,000 people) into which districts are divided. In discussing services provided at this level we will, whenever possible, designate the specific administrative subdivision, such as the "subdistrict office," that provides the service. We will continue to use the term "residents' committee" in describing the organization and services below the neighborhood level and the term "group" in describing the most local level of organization.

In June 1980, 59,000 people lived in the Fengsheng Neighborhood. The population had increased 10 percent from its 1972 level due to the excess of births over deaths and to the return of a large number of young people from the rural areas. The primary schools, which were under the administration of the neighborhood committee during the late 1960s and 1970s, are now controlled by the Bureau of Education at the district level. The Fengsheng Neighborhood Hospital and the lane health stations, which were also under the direction of the neighborhood, are now under the management of the Bureau of Public Health at the district level. Of the three nurseries to serve preschool children, two are run by residents' committees and one by Division of Preschool Children of the subdistrict; the two kindergartens are run by the subdistrict. The six factories which were previously under neighborhood auspices are now the responsibility of the municipal level of government; six new factories and twenty workshops (presumably less profitable ones) are currently under the subdistrict's administration. While residents clearly have less control today over their own schools, hospitals, and other basic services, the personnel providing these services have the benefit of professional guidance, supervision, quality control, and ongoing training.

In 1980 the neighborhood organization was divided into three parts: the Committee of the Communist Party, the General Administrative Committee (the subdistrict branch office), and the Production and Service Department. The latter two groups are under the leadership of the Committee of the Communist Party. One hundred and nineteen people work in neighborhood level administration in Fengsheng. Twenty-two people work in the Production and Service Department, which oversees the work of the local factories and workshops. Twenty-seven people work in the Subdistrict Committee of the Communist Party, which is generally concerned with administrative tasks, educating Party members, and other Party-related issues. It is also concerned with the training of members of the militia, young people, both men and women, who are organized in local factories and government offices; it is concerned with the Communist Youth League, the Women's Federation, and with the construction of air raid shelters. Yet another, albeit temporary, function of the Party Committee is to reexamine the cases of those who were persecuted during the Cultural Revolution. According to members of the committee, there are approximately 500 cases in the Fengsheng Neighborhood of people who were unjustly sent to the rural areas, people whose homes were searched and whose property was removed. Current policy is that they should be repaid in cash and goods for their damages.

The General Administrative Committee, also called the subdistrict branch office, has a staff of seventy workers who have ten major areas of responsibility: supervising the work of the twenty-six residents' committees (since 1972 Fengsheng has one additional building for government employees); urban construction, sanitation, and mobilizing the population for health work; civil adminstration, including issues of marriage and divorce; dealing with retired workers and overseas Chinese; providing employment for new middle-school graduates; family planning; preschool education; "spare-time" education (primarily for adults and young people waiting for employment); "extra-curricular" education (after-school activities); and secretarial work.

The task of providing work for middle-school graduates—both those who have recently returned from the rural areas and recent graduates—is a serious problem in China today. After the fall of the Gang of Four, young people began to return in large numbers from the countryside, where they had been sent prior to and during the Cultural Revolution. According to official Chinese estimates, approximately 17 million young people were sent from the cities to the countryside between 1968 and 1978. By the end of that decade roughly 10 million were still working in the rural areas; the remaining 7 million had been reassigned to work or study elsewhere.[9] At the National Conference on Educated Youth Settling in the Countryside, which met during the fall of 1978, the program of sending urban youths to the countryside was officially modified. The political goals were, for the most part, put to rest and the limited number of young people who would still be sent to the countryside would now go because they were explicitly surplus urban labor.

Now, of course, work must be found for the students who graduate from middle school each year. Part of the problem stems from the fact that over six million students graduated from middle school in 1980, three million took the college entrance examination and only 285,000 were admitted.[10] While the young people not accepted into college are waiting for jobs they may study at spare-time schools or technical training centers. Xinhua News Agency reported in May 1980 that approximately 8,900 jobless young people in the Chongwen District of Peking attended such programs. The same year, it was reported that over 25,000 young people were waiting for jobs in Harbin.[11]

A variety of methods are being used to alleviate the problem of unemployment among young people. In addition to obtaining work in state-owned enterprises, young people are being urged to look for work in collective units and in neighborhood-run factories. Moreover, older urban workers, particularly women, are being urged to retire at age 50 and thereby enable their children to replace them on the job.[12]

The leaders of the Fengsheng Neighborhood estimated in 1980 that they had 700 unemployed people out of approximately 35,000 working-age people, or about 2 percent unemployment. Some people were working part-time in local factories and workshops; approximately 500 young people were employed by the Production and Service Department. There is, however, considerable dissatisfaction among those working in local units. Most young people feel that they are not fully employed unless they are working in state-owned factories, in part because there are significant advantages such as higher wages and free medical care to those who work in state-owned enterprises.

The family planning activities of the subdistrict branch office have been particularly active during this current period. Two full-time workers are in charge of overall family planning programs for the entire population in the subdistrict, both those who work there and those who live there. Places of work are responsible for their employees, and residents' committees are responsible for the couples of "childbearing age" who live within their boundaries, but since 1976 an entire network has been organized to work at every level.

The functions of the organizational level below the neighborhood (subdistrict)—the residents' committees—have changed minimally since they were first established in the early 1950s. The Da Cheng Residents' Committee, for example, which includes 520 households and a population of over 1,800 people, has five primary tasks: maintenance of "social order and security," "women's work," environmental sanitation and family planning, extracurricular education for primary and secondary school students, and mediation. As part of their work in "social order and security," residents' committee members work to prevent theft and damage from "hooligans." During the Cultural Revolution, according to local cadres, schoolchildren fought and "took things from people." To counteract this behavior, residents' committee members are organizing special education for adolescents in the schools, the neighborhood, and the family. "Women's work" involves educating the woman if there is a disagreement between a husband and a wife, promoting unity between mothers-in-law and daughters-in-law, and teaching mothers how to educate their children. Comparable "men's work" does not seem to exist. Mediation includes settling disputes between neighbors, marital partners, and members of different genera-tions living in the same household. Mediation is a central function of residents' committees; in 1979, for example, residents' committees in Peking mediated 43,683 cases of civil disputes, five times as many cases as were handled that year by the district people's courts.[13] The Da Cheng Residents' Committee has seven paid full-time workers, elected by the residents. During the summer of 1980 citywide elections took place in Peking's more than 2,000 residents' committees; each commit-tee then elects its director and deputy-directors who then must be approved by the subdistrict.[14]

In the words of one member of the Fengsheng Subdistrict Office, the local committees are currently concerned with "problems of daily life." They continue to provide a two-way channel of communication from the district level to the general population; to mobilize the popu-lation to support local, regional, and national policies; and to provide, often informally, human services that people in other societies must rely on professionals to provide. These local groups have in the past few years, however, lost control of certain professional and quasi-professional services and have lost a certain amount of fiscal autonomy.

Mental Health Services

The family, the community, and the workplace play a significant role in helping people to deal with their emotional problems. The organization of life in China's neighborhoods and place of work can perhaps best be viewed as a total community support system, one largely fostered and maintained by the residents and workers them-selves. This system encourages people to see themselves as part of a total social structure, inspires them to participate actively in that social structure, and comes to their aid during times of stress.

Most people, furthermore, belong to small groups (*xiaozu*) in which both personal and public issues are discussed. If an individual has a problem in his or her personal or work life, that problem will, in all likelihood, be discussed at a meeting of the group. These small groups are characterized by a level of intimacy rarely shared in urban America outside of, perhaps, certain therapy groups. One American who has lived in China for several years has observed that study groups are composed of people with whom one works every day or of neighbors whose life is intimately linked to one's own and that everyone is well versed in the others' personalities and traits. This intimacy and interdependence continues outside of study groups and pervades much of Chinese life. The availability of these informal means of solving problems works to minimize the number of problems that actually come before the formal mental-health-care system.

Many of the social values and key innovations observable in Chinese society are also prominent features of contemporary Chinese psychiatric practice: sharing of responsibility between lay people and medical personnel in the identification, prevention, and treatment of mental illness; the subordination of individual interests for the common good; and the faith in human ability to modify individual behavior and the environment.[15] Much of what the West considers to be mental illness is handled at the neighborhood or residents' committee level in the cities or at the brigade level in the countryside. At these levels, interpersonal disputes and minor diseases, including some psychosomatic illness, are handled by paraprofessionals (Red Cross Health Workers or barefoot doctors), elected representatives with no special training for this work, or cadres. As we have seen, the people who work at these tasks are chosen because of their personal qualities, because they are seen as community activists or indigenous leaders, and because they are frequently seen as skillful mediators. When emotional problems are clearly beyond the scope of these workers, the individual may be referred to commune or county hospitals in the rural areas or psychiatric prevention stations at the district level in the cities.

Long before Western psychiatric theories entered Chinese medical thinking there were two divergent streams of thought that explained mental illness: the philosophical or medical approach, and folk beliefs and folk medical practices. Both theories have had great impact on modern Chinese psychiatric thinking.

As discussed in chapter two, ancient Chinese medical writings attributed all disease, including mental illness, to an imbalance of two forces: the *yin* and the *yang*. This imbalance was thought to be caused by deviation from the *dao*, the "way," which provided the guide for all morality and human conduct. The *dao* can be further thought of as being an "ethical superstructure"; once transgression against this ethical superstructure occurred, return to health was through a return to *dao*.[16]

While there was no supernatural element in the philosophical or medical explanation, the popular or folk beliefs about the origins of mental illness were based almost entirely on supernatural causes. And while the believers in *dao* saw the mind and the body as indivisible, popular belief considered the mind and the body as separate entities. Spirits and demons were thought from earliest times to be responsible for many of the ills that befell people.

Once a demon or spirit entered persons and made them ill it needed to be exorcised. The first exorcists were members of a priest-hood called *wu*, which to the present day has the meaning of wizard, witch, expeller of demons. *Wu* is first encountered in the *Rites of the Zhou Dynasty* (1122–244 B.C.), and it came eventually to be synonymous with the word for physician, *wuyi*, meaning "magical physician."[17] Since the mentally ill person was thought to be possessed by a spirit or demon, the onset of illness was swift. The cure might be equally sudden since the *wu*, by his ministrations, could exorcise the demon quickly. Swift exorcism led to a belief in the curability of mental illness that seems to have been carried through to the present. There was, however, a long history of stigmatization of mental illness in China before 1949.

The first mental hospital was opened in Guangzhou (Canton) in 1897. Although it started with only thirty beds and increased in size to 500 beds, it was closed in the 1930s.[18] The first academic division of neurology was established at Peking Union Medical College in 1921, the year it was founded, as part of the Department of Medicine; a Department of Psychiatry and Neurology was established at PUMC in 1932.

The growth of psychiatry and neurology in China up to 1949 was very slow, however.[19]

In 1949 there were four psychiatric hospitals in all of China: Peking, Shanghai, Guangzhou, and Nanjing. Other psychiatric beds were located in general hospitals in the larger coastal cities. All told, there were between 1,000 and 6,000 beds. The best treatment available was custodial care, although the majority of patients were bound to their beds, kept in filthy conditions, and often physically abused. For most mentally ill people, there was no treatment at all; they were either kept isolated at home or roamed the streets.[20]

Mental health was not given high priority in the early years of the People's Republic, although some of the initial health campaigns such as those to eradicate venereal disease, opium addiction, and prostitution certainly had profound effects on the Chinese people's mental health. Additional facilities were established, so that by 1957 the number of psychiatric beds had been increased to 20,000. Psychiatric services spread at an even greater rate in the late 1950s and early 1960s. Before the Cultural Revolution, all medical schools had courses in psychiatry, and neuropsychiatric research was carried on widely. During the early 1960s traditional medicine—including acupuncture, breathing exercises, and the use of herb medicine—and Western medicine, including insulin shock and electroshock, were used in the treatment of mental disease.

During the Cultural Revolution period there was increased emphasis in psychiatric practice, as in all branches of medicine, on combining the techniques of traditional and Western medicine. The use of electroshock and insulin shock treatments was discontinued and Western-trained doctors revamped their psychiatric services to include a greater emphasis on traditional methods and on political techniques adopted by the society at large. The major methods used during the early 1970s included drug therapy, acupuncture, "heart-to-heart talks," group discussions, productive labor, follow-up care, and the teachings of Chairman Mao.

Another concept that was widely used during the Cultural Revolution period was "revolutionary optimism." Revolutionary optimism places the patient and his or her immediate problems in broad historical perspective. The patient is seen above all as part of the revolution, and the revolution, it is felt, will surely be victorious. Thus, no matter what the difficulties, "the patient will have a bright future." Patients are urged to obtain treatment and overcome their illness not only for their own sake but also for the sake of the revolution. Revolutionary optimism gives patients the encouragement and confidence to conquer their disease. Although the Chinese did not specifically discuss it, nationalism is a key component of revolutionary optimism; working for a better China and being a part of the revolution in China are implicit in the ideology.

Another aspect of revolutionary optimism is the recognition that one's own problems pale in comparison with those of people who have sacrificed themselves for the revolution. Doctors at the Peking Medical College told of patients suffering from neuroses who are taught that others with even greater hardships are nevertheless struggling to overcome them for the good of the revolution. They are told of members of the People's Liberation Army who have been seriously wounded but still bravely struggle against their wounds, of workers in Shanghai who suffered burns over 90 percent of their bodies but still try to overcome their illness, of pilots who have lost both legs but work effectively with their prostheses. An old man lost his son during the war of Liberation, and was "very sad." He was told that there were thousands of people who made such sacrifices during the war of Liberation. Even in Chairman Mao's family, he was told, there were many people killed. The patient was in this way encouraged to "handle his feelings correctly"; he "changed his sorrow into strength, his low spirit into high spirit."

Another integral component of revolutionary optimism was the subordination of one's own feelings to the cause of the revolution. As Oksenberg has written of the Chinese revolutionary view of the New Man: "Losing his old individual identity, he partakes of the greater spirit of the group and thereby achieves a spiritual transformation."[21]

A recent evaluation from China of developments during the late 1960s and first half of the 1970s states that "during this period the influence of ultra-left ideology interfered greatly with Chinese psychiatry." The article, published in the *Chinese Medical Journal*, continues:

> In these years, work was done on only two aspects. Most provinces, cities, regions and districts carried out epidemiologic psychiatric investigations, psychiatric workers leaving the hospitals to make

social investigations and spreading mental health know-how and serving the people on the spot.

With the help of local administrative units and the people, they set up a prevention and treatment network. Traditional Chinese medicine including proven prescriptions, acupuncture and moxibustion was used extensively. However, as little attention was paid to research design and experimental methodology few reports of academic value were written despite thousands of people being investigated epidemiologically and hundreds and thousands being treated.[22]

It is exceedingly difficult to estimate the amount of mental illness in China at present. There are no nationwide data available and only limited data are available for large urban centers. Furthermore, since mental illness is largely viewed by the Chinese as equivalent to psychosis and still apparently carries a certain amount of stigma for the families involved, it may be handled within the family unit or within the production brigade in the rural areas or the residents' committee in the urban areas. Furthermore, there is evidence from the investigations of some Western scientists into the incidence of mental illness in China that much of what would be labeled mental illness in the West is seen as somatic illness in China and treated as such.[23]

Surveys of Peking, Shanghai, Nanjing, and other major cities in 1978 were reported by the Ministry of Health to show a rate of "mental illness" of 5 to 7 per 1,000 and of "serious mental illness" of 2 to 4 per 1,000. Statistics for Peking released in 1980 indicate that the city's mental hospitals have a total of 2,500 beds for a population of seven million, one bed for every 3,000 people. According to these estimates, 5.6 of every 1,000 people of Peking are patients in the mental health system. These are said not to include cases of neurosis. Efforts are being made to treat mental patients in their homes rather than in institutions, and to this end "mental illness clinics" and prevention and treatment centers have been established in Peking.[24]

Most people who enter hospitals as mental patients are helped to make the decision themselves by family, friends, and co-workers. In the rare cases where patients are not in a condition to make this judgment for themselves, the family will have the patient committed. The patient is encouraged to see the problem not as a personal failing, but as an illness that needs care. In addition, the patient's job is kept open and he or she is given full pay while hospitalized.

Medication is used to help the patient achieve a state where psychotherapy and other activities can be undertaken. The medications include chlorpromazine (Thorazine), used in smaller doses than in the West, phenothiazines, and antidepressants. Insulin shock and electroshock therapy are being used once again. Whenever possible herbal medications are substituted for Western medications in order to avoid undesirable side effects and to reduce costs. Acupuncture is widely used both to calm anxious, overexcited patients and to stimulate depressed patients.

Physical exercise is considered an important adjunct to treatment, as is some form of physical labor. Mental patients contribute to the maintenance of the institution by performing various types of jobs, from working with the herbal medications to gardening and growing their own vegetables. They also do jobs on consignment from local factories.

While these aspects of treatment are essential, they are seen as adjuncts to the main focus of treatment, which is psychotherapy. The medications and/or acupuncture treatments are methods to get the patient into a frame of mind where it is possible to engage in psychotherapy. The therapy itself consists of several different forms, individual therapy, which is called "heart-to-heart talks," and group sessions.

The average stay in a mental hospital is two to three months; hospitalization lasting as long as a year has been reported, but such instances are said to be rare. Patients who cannot be returned to the community may be referred to large chronic disease hospitals, which the Chinese refer to as sanatoriums. These are frequently under the auspices of large factories and state-run industries that provide care for chronic mental illness and other chronic diseases.[25] When a patient is ready for discharge, medical workers visit the community and workplace to prepare the patient's friends, relatives, and co-workers with an understanding of his problems. If it is thought that the former job of the patient contributed to his mental problems, another job within the same workplace is found.

Since 1976 activities in the field of psychiatry have proliferated: psychiatric journals have begun publishing again, national conferences have been held, and research efforts have been greatly expanded. Hospital-based postgraduate courses have been organized in several cities and international exchange in the field of psychiatry has increased significantly. As the Chinese themselves state, "Chinese psychiatry is a developing field," and while they are open to ideas from other countries they clearly emphasize that "China has its own culture, customs, . . . habits, and social system" and therefore needs to use "the best experience of other countries combined with China's concrete conditions."[26]

Social Welfare Services

Social welfare benefits are provided to those in need through a variety of administrative units. China's policy of decentralization has meant that responsibility for aspects of human services such as health, education, and welfare has been placed in the hands of neighborhoods, factories and communes. Each administrative unit has been encouraged to develop its own social service system. Consequently, inequities have developed between urban and rural areas and within the rural sector. China's major technique to minimize these inequities has been the transfer of personnel from the cities to the countryside; the "sending down" of educated youth was also a mechanism for promoting greater equality between the two sectors.

In the rural areas those in need may receive assistance from the production teams' or brigades' welfare fund. This category is quite small since both the 1950 and the 1981 Marriage Laws stipulate that "children have the duty to support and assist their parents."[27] Those households which need to be supported by the society are usually composed of the chronically ill who cannot work, childless widows or widowers, or orphans. There are basically two types of care for childless elderly persons: the first is the institutional "homes for the respected aged" and the second is the "five-guarantee household." Under the former arrangement, the elderly person moves out of his or her home and into the institution to be cared for and supported by the public welfare fund. Under the second arrangement, the elderly person remains in his or her own home, is cared for by relatives or friends, and the five basic needs (food, clothing, shelter, medical care, and decent burial) are provided by the collective.[28] Local welfare funds are also available to those who are in debt to the collective, usually due to receiving more advances in grain than they are entitled to.

There is no old-age social insurance in China except for employees in government-owned enterprises. Men may retire at the age of 60, women at the age of 50 or 55, and for workers in dangerous occupations (such as mines and quarries) retirement is five years earlier. Pensions range from 60 percent to 90 percent of one's last wage level, depending on length of service; the maximum pension is reached after 20 years of work for men and 15 years of work for women. "Model workers" and old revolutionaries are entitled to higher pensions.[29] A pension of 60 to 75 percent of the previous wages is provided for those with work-related injuries resulting in complete disability.

China's elderly, orphans, severely handicapped, and mentally retarded who have no one to care for them are supported by social welfare benefits provided by the state. The state annually allocates funds for this purpose. There are now 500 social welfare institutions and 200 homes for the aged providing care for approximately 60,000 people in China's cities.

The Changzhi welfare center in Shanxi Province in North China is an example of an institution which provides care for handicapped people. The center was organized in 1954 and currently cares for 50 deaf mutes, orphans, and blind, disabled, and mentally ill people. Those who have relatives do not live at the center and are entitled to an allowance the amount of which depends on their relatives' income. At the center, food, clothing, shelter, and medical care are free. Orphans who are not otherwise disabled only remain there until they are old enough to obtain work and care for themselves.[30]

The Chinese estimate that there are currently over 3 million deaf mutes and approximately 1.6 million blind people in China. Numerous services have been developed to improve their living conditions. The most important, perhaps, is the availability of job opportunities. Over 900 factories have been organized under local government auspices to provide employment for blind and deaf workers. The profit earned by these factories is used for the well-being of the workers.[31] These services are in striking contrast to the care of the blind prior to the revolution. The blind in China in the 1940s have been described as "isolated in a tangle of superstition, fear and contempt." Blind children might have been abandoned or sold as slaves; whatever their fate their blindness was frequently considered a punishment for their parents' or ancestors' sins.[32]

Schools for the blind and the deaf have been established throughout China. Before Liberation there were only 3,000 students enrolled in 41 such schools; today there are 32,000 students enrolled in over 290 schools.[33] In addition, part-work part-study schools, technical and professional schools, and spare-time evening schools have been organized to meet their needs.

A publishing house for the blind publishes five periodicals and a large variety of books in braille. In 1954 the China Blind People's Welfare Institute and in 1956 the China Welfare Institute of the Deaf were founded; both of these groups are mass organizations with local branches. During the Cultural Revolution the work of these organizations was discontinued, but local branches have been reorganized during the last few years.

The Chinese feel that they lag behind industrialized societies in their work with the blind and the deaf, particularly with regard to educational opportunities. Organized preschool education for them is nonexistent. Most of the schools are for primary school students, but not all blind and deaf children are in school. Middle and technical schools are relatively rare. In addition, there are no institutes in all of China to train teachers for this special population.

In the future the Chinese plan to provide universal primary school education and to train special teachers to teach the blind and the deaf. They hope to provide even greater work opportunities and plan to concentrate greater resources on prevention, treatment, and research on these problems.

The Shanghai Children's Welfare Institute, originally an orphanage run by missionaries prior to 1949, is now administered by the Shanghai Municipal Affairs Bureau and cares for approximately 500 patients, most of whom range in age from newborns to age sixteen. The Institute cares primarily for three groups of children: handicapped children from infancy to three years, educable children who range in age from three to sixteen, and severely retarded children for whom the emphasis is on training rather than on education.[34] Included in these three groups is a group of 76 handicapped children who were not served by this institution prior to 1979, children who have family members who could take care of them. According to the Director, Yang Jiezeng, the Institute accepts these children to ease the burden on the parents. By relieving their problems at home, the Institute enables the parents to work without constant worry about their child. These parents are urged to bring their children home for weekends and holidays, are given regular reports on their children's condition, and are invited to observe the training the children receive and to participate in the training themselves. The cost to the parents is 20 yuan per month including full-time care and food.

The children who are considered educable include deaf mutes and blind children who have normal intelligence; they live at the Institute but are sent out to special schools. Another group includes those who also have normal intelligence and a minor handicap; they attend a regular school nearby. Those who have normal intelligence and a severe handicap and those who are of preschool and kindergarten age are educated at the Institute. There is, in addition, one retarded group of children who are being educated at the Institute through experimental methods stressing such imitative activities as singing and dancing.

The severely disabled and retarded group who comprise 120 of the total number of children at the Institute are generally unable to care for themselves when they are first admitted. They are gradually taught to sit, stand, walk, and eventually eat by themselves.

According to Dr. Li Qingshu, the physician in charge of medical work, doctors in a wide variety of subspecialities work with the children. Following a child's admission there is a forty-day period of observation after which the decision is made about which group he or she should be placed in. The children suffer from a variety of illnesses: diseases of the central nervous system (27 percent), endocrine disease (2 percent), chromosome deformity (4 percent), mental retardation from unknown causes (38 percent), musculoskeletal disease (8 percent), diseases of the ears, nose, and throat (13 percent), cardiorenal disease (4 percent), dermatological disease (1 percent), and miscellaneous (3 percent).

Many of the children in this institution had been abandoned—in waiting rooms in a hospital, in railway stations, on the docks or the street early in the morning. They were abandoned, personnel believe, because of the parents' superstitious ideas about handicapped and retarded children. Such children are often viewed as monsters or ghosts, as foreign spirits that have come to the parents as punishment for something they have done. These views are particularly widespread in the countryside. The social welfare workers try to find the parents to explain their child's illness to them and to explain what they can do to help them.

Another group housed in the Institute are 67 elderly people who have no relatives to care for them. Some are ill; some are simply retired workers who have a pension to pay for their food and rent. In order to be accepted they must apply and meet the conditions for admission. They then visit the Institute and, if they are satisfied with what they find, may decide to accept the place offered. They are free to come and go as they like and interact with the children on a voluntary basis.

The broad goal of the Institute is to enable as many children as possible to learn to care for themselves and live and work in the larger society. Children who cannot live on their own after age sixteen are transferred to the Shanghai Second Welfare Institute. The other goal that is stressed is prevention; the medical personnel are currently concentrating on tracing family histories and other research in order to minimize the number of cases in the future.

The Institute's cost for providing care for these children is 60 yuan per child per month and the total operating funds, 30,000 yuan per month (excluding the cost of new equipment), are provided by the Shanghai municipality.

As we have seen, since the Chinese Communist Party assumed power in 1949 it has experimented with a number of techniques for governing and providing services to the cities. While the Chinese government has utilized the dual approach of reliance on bureaucracy and mass participation, the emphasis on each has varied considerably, depending on the then-current emphasis in political ideology. The stress on antielitism and popular participation during the Cultural Revolution period was reflected in the cities in increased power at the local level. The current stress on rapid modernization, efficient management, and increased production is reflected in the dismantling of neighborhood revolutionary committees and the resumption of administrative control by the district. Mass participation remains nevertheless an important aspect of urban life at the residents' committee level, where activists are concerned with "problems of daily life" rather than administrative and financial control.

In addition to services provided locally by nonprofessional, indigenous leaders, the Chinese have developed limited professional services for the mentally ill, the handicapped, the deaf, and the blind. While these services have been significantly expanded since Liberation, the Chinese are the first to state that they are grossly inadequate. It is expected that in the future more attention will be paid to the training of professionals to serve this population and to increased development of services at all levels.

6 | The Family and Child Care: The First Collective

Family Structure

The Chinese peasant prior to Liberation lived under a dual oppression: the semifeudal economic system and the traditional family system. Both were based on a hierarchy of domination and subservience that was enforced at all levels with brutality and violence. William Hinton in his book *Fanshen* describes this hierarchy of violence: "Husbands beat their wives, mothers-in-law beat their daughters-in-law, peasants beat their children, [and] landlords beat their tenants."[1] Although traditional family and village life contained elements of mutual caring, there was omnipresent exploitation by the government, the war lords, landlords, husbands, and mothers-in-law of the peasant, his wife, and their children.

The family life of both peasants and gentry was governed as well by a highly structured authoritarian system. All family members had their place "in proper order by their age," and respect for the older members, chronologically and in generation, was a basic principle of life. The kinship system was based on three factors: generation, age, and proximity of kinship. One's place in the system was determined and fixed.

Relationships between parents and children were based on the dual principles of filial piety and veneration of age. As the peasants were completely subservient to the landlords, so were the children completely subservient to the parents. Filial piety was enhanced by genuine affection between parents and their children, and these emotional bonds were further strengthened by the interdependence of parents and children. Parents were dependent on their sons for security in their old age; children were dependent on their parents for survival. The existence of children was threatened from all sides. Infanticide was legal, physical abuse was rife, and the peasants were powerless to assure their children's, as well as their own, basic necessities.

The superior position of the male in pre–Liberation China is evident. The purpose of marriage was to produce male heirs to perpetuate the paternal grandparents' family, assure the continuity of the husband's family structure, and provide additional work power from the son and daughter-in-law. According to one historian of pre–revolutionary China, "A man who had no sons was considered to be childless . . . If, indeed, a boy was born the whole family rejoiced, but if a girl arrived everyone was dejected. On the third day after her birth it was the custom to place a girl on the floor beneath her bed, and to make her grasp a tile and a pebble so that even then she would begin to form a lifelong habit of submission and an acquaintance with hardship. In contrast, in early times when a boy was born arrows were shot from an exorcising bow in the four directions of the compass and straight up and down."[2]

In addition to having their feet bound, women were kept to their menial role by a number of other practices. While illiteracy was generally high in China before Liberation, women were denied an education even more systematically than men. Women were not permitted to take the civil service examinations and thus were excluded a priori from becoming officials and, even more important, from the primary route out of a life of manual labor. In addition to being denied education, women were discouraged from developing any skills outside those related to the home or from working outside the home. They would thus be completely dependent economically on their husbands and on their in-laws, no matter how badly they were treated.

In all social classes, both urban or rural, women were married at a young age to men they were not likely to know beforehand. Marriages were arranged by both sets of parents, with a view to strengthening the family of the groom. The young bride moved to her in-laws' home, belonged to her husband's family, and was discouraged from even visiting her own family. Essentially, she lost her identity as a human being and was totally subservient to the needs and wishes of her new family. Most of all, she was a slave to her mother-in-law, who, similarly enslaved for years by her mother-in-law, perpetuated the tradition.

Women were married for life; they were not permitted to divorce. Even when the husband died, remarriage was frowned upon, for the widow was still considered part of her husband's family. Suicide was the only way out of her miserable existence, and female suicides were not uncommon in the old China.

Women's role and the traditional Chinese family were not transformed suddenly after Liberation in 1949. From the turn of the century until the Revolution of 1911, Western ideas of equality for women and a less authoritarian family structure gradually penetrated the Chinese intellectual community. In 1911, with the overthrow of the Emperor and the rise to power of Sun Yat-sen, women's right to education was promulgated and women were encouraged to marry voluntarily and to participate in government. Following the Republican revolution, the New Culture movement of 1917 and the May 4 movement of 1919 encouraged greater questioning of the traditional family, asked for a new role for women in the family as well as in society in general, and called for voluntary marriage and for greater freedom for young people.

During the 1920s women gained greater political power and, in fact, became political workers in both the Kuomintang and the Communist Party. In 1924 the Kuomintang Party called for sex equality in law, economic matters, education, and society in general. From the 1920s on, sex equality was accepted by the urban intelligentsia. With increased industrialization in the 1920s, '30s, and '40s, employment for many urban women became available in factories, women became economic assets, and consequently were accorded more respect.

During the years 1938–1945, major changes were being made in the structure of the family in the liberated areas, especially in the areas wrested from Japanese control by the Eighth Route Army. The Communist Party and the Eighth Route Army were committed to the equality of women. As they entered a village in the 1940s, one of their first acts was to organize a women's association and to encourage women to share their oppression with one another in meetings that came to be known as "Speak Bitterness" sessions.[3] During this period women were to become some of the most ardent supporters of the Communist revolution.

The abolition of the landlord system and the turning over of the land to the peasants greatly weakened the authority of the traditional Chinese family but did not eradicate the values it represented. The Communists in their 1950 Marriage Law, one of the first major laws of the new government, abolished arranged marriages; outlawed paying any price in money or goods for a wife; outlawed polygamy, concubines, and child marriage; prohibited interference in the remarriage of widows; and guaranteed the right of divorce to the wife as well as to the husband.

After the promulgation of the new Marriage Law, the Communist government placed special emphasis in their campaigns on raising the literacy of women. Classes were organized in the urban areas and in the rural areas as well. But the key factor in the liberation of women was work. In the mid-1950s, the system of work points was introduced into the rural cooperatives. Although a woman worked and earned points and was paid according to how much she worked, hard manual labor accrued more work points; therefore, men earned more points than women. Furthermore, remuneration was made to the family rather than to the individual, thereby maintaining the interdependence of family members. With the establishment of communes in 1958, women had their first real chance at equality.

Women now receive equal pay for equal work (although hard manual labor still merits more work points than lighter manual labor) and are, therefore, not as dependent upon their families or their husbands as they once were. But the role of women is closely linked to the economy; when employment drops, women workers are the first to be laid off. The liberation of women, therefore, has been inextricably tied to the fluctuation of employment in China since 1949. While women work in a wide variety of jobs and seem to have gained a significant amount of power at the local administrative level, the number of women drops sharply at higher levels of government and Party structure.

The Chinese family today is most often three-generational; the most common pattern is still for the young couple to move into the husband's parents' home. Since virtually all women under retirement age work outside the home, grandparents play an important role in child-rearing and homemaking. In fact, the Chinese family can best be viewed as a minimutual aid group in which, as the Chinese say, the old take care of the young and the middle-aged take care of the old. But while the elderly have retained much of the respect that was traditionally accorded to them, they do not have the unquestioned power they once had.

The vast majority of Chinese people marry, usually in their early to midtwenties, and the divorce rate seems to be exceedingly low. A new Marriage Law which went into effect on January 1, 1981, stipulates that although later marriage should be encouraged the minimum age for marriage is currently 22 for men and 20 for women, that marriage must be completely voluntary, and that husband and wife should enjoy equal status in the home. It also maintains the mutal responsibility of family members by stating that parents are responsible for rearing and educating their children and that children are responsible for supporting and assisting their parents.

In addition, the new law stipulates that divorce should be granted if one party insists, in cases of "complete alienation" or when mediation has failed; this is a change from the 1950 law which did not require the automatic granting of divorce in those cases. Divorce is now becoming somewhat more widespread because of these new regulations, especially in Chinese cities. The new law, following the pattern of the old law, states that the husband may not apply for a divorce while his wife is pregnant or within one year after the birth of a child.[4]

Although both the 1950 and the 1981 Marriage Laws state, "Marriage must be based upon the complete willingness of the two parties. Neither party shall use compulsion and no third party is allowed to interfere," and "The exaction of money or gifts in connection with marriage is prohibited," there is evidence that arranged marriages and the exchange of money or gifts remain widespread, particularly in the rural areas. In urban areas marriage is commonly based on love and mutual attraction but in the countryside it is more difficult for young people to meet and get to know one another.

In some rural areas a go-between introduces the two sets of parents; the parents then "consider how many members in each family share the family income and property, how many people in each family can work, and its annual income before they ask their children's opinion." If after the couple meet the man is satisfied with the match, he will leave a gift, usually money; if the woman accepts the gift, they are engaged. A survey of two rural counties in Anhui Province in 1979 indicated that of the 14,586 marriages studied, 15 percent were by free choice, 75 percent were arranged but agreed to by the couple, and 10 percent were arranged only by the parents.[5]

Marriage arrangements appear to be less dependent on the parents in the cities. In urban areas young people may meet with the aid of a Marriage Introduction Service such as the one affiliated with the Shanghai Shipping Bureau. Interested individuals fill out a question-naire, attaching a photograph, and the Service attempts to introduce single people to one another.

Getting married in revolutionary China is not inexpensive. A recent survey of a typical village in the North China province of Hebei indicates that it costs an average young peasant male 3,000 yuan to marry, most of that money earmarked for building a three-room home and buying furniture. Betrothal gifts and the wedding banquet will cost the groom's family at least another 1,000 yuan. After the engage-ment, the young man is expected to give his fiancée money for new clothes and sometimes a wristwatch, a bicycle, and a washing machine. In Peking a television set, it is said, has become de rigueur. Considering the fact that the average peasant in China only earns from 100 to 400 yuan per year and the average beginning worker earns approximately 50 yuan per month these gifts clearly represent a hardship for young men and their families.

While there have been efforts to democratize relationships within the family and to move away from rigid role differentiation—men are being encouraged to participate in housework and child-rearing as women have been encouraged to work outside the home—there is also substantial evidence that the revolution has actually strengthened a "reformed version of the traditional peasant family." According to a recent analysis of the modern Chinese family, "Patrilocality, a semi-arranged marriage system, and even a form of bride-price appear to be durable survivals in postrevolutionary rural China. There are a variety of indications that . . . this modified traditional family system and the muted version of patriarchy that it supports, are strong, stable and remarkably unquestioned in the People's Republic of China."[6]

Furthermore, the potential consequences of the new responsibility system in the rural areas on the role of women are as yet unclear. The establishment of an individual work point system at the time the communes were organized in the late 1950s provided women with independently determined income. Each worker, rather than each household, earned work points based on the kind and amount of work he or she performed. Women were therefore not necessarily economically tied to their husbands. Under the new responsibility system, the household as a unit contracts with the production team to farm a specific amount of land and to meet specific production quotas. It is ironic that while the Chinese are moving from collective responsibility for farming the land to individual household responsibility, they are at the same time moving from individual income calculation within the collective commune structure to income calculation for the household as a unit.

The production team negotiates with the head of the household (who is very likely to be the male adult) and, from published reports of areas in which the responsibility system has been tried, income and produce are earned by the household as a single unit rather than by individuals within the household. Will this system, if widely adopted, tie women even more closely to their husbands? Will they, once again, be working under their husbands' authority? What will be the economic options for women who may wish to divorce their husbands?

The new responsibility system may, in addition, be in direct conflict with China's intensive drive to lower the birth rate. A household with several children would appear to have an even clearer economic advantage over one with the strongly recommended single child.

Preschool Care

The socialization process in China has, both in traditional and in modern times, included formal education as a key element. In traditional China, however, the educational system taught significantly different attitudes and roles to the elite than it did to the peasantry. In pre-revolutionary China the educational ladder and examination system provided the possibility of a government job and public respect while the study of Confucian classics provided a guide to personal conduct and correct behavior.[7] Confucianism taught the scholars and gentry to develop a sound moral character, take care of family affairs, set one's kingdom in order, and bring peace to the empire.[8] The common people, particularly the peasants, were also expected to be guided by formal Confucian teaching but were only expected to observe the first two steps. Consequently a social order developed "in which the scholars and the gentry constituted a national-minded minority, while the majority of the common people confined themselves largely to individual and family affairs without knowledge of the greater community and national interest and without any deep sense of moral obligation to it."[9] In short, while the elite were expected to be concerned with both public and private issues, the common people were expected to limit their concerns to private matters.

During the 1930s and 1940s, the Chinese Communists in the remote border areas and in the Yan'an base attempted to develop educational policies that would be functional within their situation of nearly constant warfare and would aid in their desperate need to develop production. By 1944 experimental educational programs in Yan'an stressed spreading literacy quickly and teaching practical economic skills. Under the slogan "Develop production, expand the schools," new schools, including night schools, literacy groups tied to production units, and half-time schools, were established for the part-time education of peasants and workers. Reflecting the Chinese preoccupation with mass participation, "the 1944 education goals envisioned nothing less than the participation of every man, woman and child in the educational process."[10] The Chinese Communist Party hoped to transform within one generation the great mass of illiterate peasants, through their direct participation in society, from feudal thinking characterized by superstition, fatalism, and passivity to a modern scientific outlook characterized by reason, optimism, and commitment to the larger society.

After they took power in 1949, the Chinese Communists used a variety of techniques to transform the thinking and the ideology of their massive population. They utilized radio broadcasts, films, operas, ballet, posters, and printed materials, but primarily they used formal education and interaction within small groups. The formal educational system in China since 1949 has attempted to transmit both general knowledge and specific technical skills to facilitate modernization, and simultaneously through a variety of forms—literacy classes in the early 1950s, part-time school for workers, refresher courses for all levels of professionals, and through the primary, secondary, and university systems—it has encouraged the population to take an active role in their society, feel a broad commitment to the country as a whole, and act on the basis of public rather than simply private goals.

The use of the educational system to socialize the children, to teach a system of values and attitudes, is perhaps most clearly observed in preschool care. Preschool education was essentially nonexistent in China prior to 1949. After 1949, and particularly at the time of the Great Leap Forward, 1957–1958, the mobilization of women into the work force led to the gradual development of nurseries and kinder-gartens for those families in which there was no grandmother or other caretaker available to care for the children. In addition to freeing mothers to participate in production, providing the children's initial educational experience, and supplying children's health care and a significant part of their nutritional requirements, preschool facilities taught the values and attitudes of the newly established revolutionary society.

In removing small children for several hours at a time from their primary group of the family and particularly from the influence of the grandmother, the most frequent alternate caretaker, the Chinese were attempting to remove them, insofar as they had appropriate personnel available, from attitudes and values which had been formed by tradi-tional Chinese society and which were frequently in conflict with newer, revolutionary values. While the family remains a strong force in China, the shifting of a significant part of the socialization process from the family unit to the community or larger society as embodied by the nursery or kindergarten was a major break with traditional Chinese society.

Chinese educational theory and practice have been derived in part from the philosophy of John Dewey and in larger part from the educa-tional philosophy and practice of the Soviet Union, which had also been influenced by progressive education. The belief in the importance of "Communist morality,"[11] the belief that education can transform human attitudes and behavior, and the belief that the child must feel identified with a series of concentric collectives of which the family is the primary one,[12] are rooted both in Marxist educational philosophy and in the extensive Soviet efforts to provide care for preschool children. Even details such as the fifty-six-day maternity leave and the policy of encouraging the children to do "productive labor" are modeled, at least in part, on the Russian experience. Chinese preschool care is, however, far less centralized and standardized than its Russian counterpart; general policy trends are developed centrally and each area is then encouraged to implement them using their own techniques.

Preschool children occupy a unique place in Chinese society. While traditionally, "Chinese parental affection toward . . . children (was) . . . both genuine and strong,"[13] the poverty under which the vast majority of Chinese people lived led not infrequently to child labor, the sale of children, and female infanticide. In recent years the preschool child has been indulged, viewed as special, not subject to the usual expectations and restrictions of the older child or adult. Preschool children's clothing, symbolic of their different status, is far more colorful and decorative than that of adults and children over the age of seven. In addition, young children are permitted considerably more behavioral leeway, are disciplined far less, and seem to be the objects of more overt warmth and physical contact than school-aged children. Nevertheless, all children, including preschool children, are considered citizens of China who have responsibilities to their society, albeit responsibilities appropriate to their age and stage of development, and therefore need to know the current political "line." Alongside this dual view of the role of children is the Maoist belief that environment, specifically including education, can fundamentally shape an individual's character and behavior. As the report of a group who visited China in 1973 observed, "The Chinese . . . have a profound faith in the ability of proper educational procedures to produce desired attitudes, values, and emotions in children."[14] In short, Mao's belief that education can "enable people to develop morally, intellectually and physically so they become 'well-educated worker(s) imbued with socialist consciousness.'"[15] has profoundly affected the nature and content of preschool care.

According to the *China Economic Yearbook* of 1981, 11,507,700 children attend 170,000 preschool facilities nationwide.[16] These numbers seem to indicate that approximately 10 to 15 percent of

China's children in the age range three to seven are cared for in pre-school facilities. According to other data from the Committee for the Defense of Children and other Chinese sources, however, approximately one fourth of the preschool children attend preschool facilities.[17]

While the estimate of 11.5 million children in preschool facilities in 1981 is significantly higher than the estimate of 8.8 million in 1979, it is lower than the estimate for 1976 published in the 1980 *China Ency-clopedia Yearbook*. In 1976, according to the yearbook, 13,955,000 students were enrolled in 443,700 preschool facilities, which are termed "kindergartens."[18] The Chinese Committee for the Defense of Children now claims that these 1976 statistics are "impossible." Leading mem-bers of the committee say that they have no accurate figures for 1976 at this time, but they offer several explanations for the discrepancy. First, they claim that during the period of the Gang of Four there was "great exaggeration" in statistics in certain fields and possibly this was the case in preschool education. Second, in the past "seasonal" kinder-gartens which were organized in the countryside during busy seasons might have been counted as full facilities; now they are not. Third, the Ministry of Education is currently attempting to register all preschool facilities and therefore both obtain a more accurate count and exert greater control over teaching, sanitary conditions, and other facets of preschool care.

The representatives of the committee emphasize the difficulty of gathering statistics on preschool facilities both before and after 1976: "Our country is so big and so widespread; how can a count like this be wholly accurate? We have many different kinds of kindergartens, not only those set up by state organizations or enterprises, but street kindergartens, kindergartens set up by other lower-level organizations, and even a few private kindergartens. We say that in China there are 300,000,000 children below the age of 14, but even that can only be an estimate. We will have to wait until the census in July of 1982 for an accurate count."

In any case, the percentage of children cared for clearly varies considerably from place to place. In the Peking Municipality, for ex-ample, 58.9 percent of the preschool population attend 6,328 nurseries and kindergartens,[19] while in Shenyang, an industrial city in the north-east, 68 percent of the city's preschool children attend 2,450 nurseries and kindergartens.[20] While adequate statistics are not available, it is clear that percentages in the rural areas are far lower. Recognizing the inadequacy of current facilities, the deputy head of the Peking Municipality's Women's Federation recently called for the development of additional nurseries and kindergartens.

Children who attend preschool facilities generally spend ten to twelve hours a day at "part-time" kindergartens; a small number attend "full-time" kindergartens twenty-four hours a day and only return home Saturday afternoon until Sunday evening or Monday morning. Furthermore, a consensus exists in China around child-rearing attitudes and practices that is rarely if ever seen in the West. Not only do the nursery and kindergarten teachers agree about promoting the "Four Modernizations," but they tend to agree on when and how to toilet train, how to treat the overly active child, and how to deal with the "naughty" child.

The basic structure of urban preschool care was established during the late 1950s and has not been altered significantly since that time. At the end of maternity leave, which usually lasts fifty-six days, an infant may be brought to a nursing room in the factory or institution where the mother works. Nursing rooms are so named because the mothers visit them twice a day to feed their babies. At approximately a year and a half the children, weaned to the cup, move from nursing rooms to nurseries in the mother's or possibly the father's place of employment and from the age of three to six or six and a half children are cared for in kindergartens, which are considerably larger and more elaborate than facilities for younger children. These are generally located in residential neighborhoods but may also be located in work units or attached to primary schools.

Preschool facilities vary enormously from sparsely furnished, informal rural nurseries and kindergartens staffed frequently by untrained older women to modern facilities in the major cities, staffed by trained, experienced teachers; the programs which will be described in this chapter are primarily in urban settings. Fees for preschool care also vary from place to place. Parents pay the cost of the food the children receive and generally pay half the cost of the tuition, the parent's work unit paying the other half. Financial arrangements in the rural areas range from a mother paying as much as one fifth of her income for preschool care to her only paying for food.

While nursery classes may have smaller numbers of children and only two teachers, the typical kindergarten class has approximately twenty-seven children and may have either two or three teachers. All of the teachers relate to all of the children, getting to know them intimately over the course of the year. Most modification of behavior is accomplished by praising the behavior the teachers wish to see repeated rather than by negative disciplinary control. Models of behavior, both fictitious and real, are also used to illustrate desirable attitudes and behavior. "Education should serve the workers. Our goal is to train children by means of socialist education and socialist culture to be the successors to the socialist cause," the "responsible member" of the Revolutionary Committee of the Beihai Kindergarten in Peking declared in 1971.[21] Every effort was made during the Cultural Revolution to inculcate "proletarian values," to teach children, in the words of another teacher, "to love the workers, peasants and soldiers" and to "serve the people."

In nursing rooms children were often placed several to a large crib or two or more to a playpen. Cooperation and collective thinking were encouraged at every stage; the children were even toilet-trained collectively. Little effort was made to stimulate the children intellectually; the focus was on caring for them and on teaching cooperation. The walls of nursing rooms were generally bare, few toys were in evidence. The care-givers, called "aunties" rather than teachers, usually had no special training and were frequently selected from among the workers in the factory who were the "most responsible and the most patient."

In the nurseries the children were encouraged to think of themselves as a minicollective and urged to heed the words from Mao Zedong's 1944 essay, "Serve the People": to "care for each other, love and help each other."[22] But their education centered not only on their interpersonal relationships and on mutual aid but also on relating their world to the wider world around them. A group of three-year-olds seated on small chairs chugged as though they were a train and sang a song about going on a train to Peking; they then turned around in their chairs and became horses riding to Peking. They finished their performance by gaily singing and dancing "Chairman Mao is Our Great Leader," with the teachers in the room singing along and tapping their feet. In these polished, enthusiastic, ubiquitous performances in the early 1970s, for which Chinese children are justly famous, the vast majority of songs and dances involved political topics. In the words of the Vice-Chairman of the Revolutionary Committee of the Da Cheng Nursery in the Fengsheng Neighborhood in Peking in 1972, "We want to teach the children to love their leader, to love their motherland, to love labor, the people and the collective [the "five loves"]. We teach them through stories and pictures, through singing revolutionary songs, through painting, and even through exercise." A group of two-and-a-half-year-olds, fulfilling the words of their teacher, sang, "The sun is red; the sun is bright; the sun shines all over like a sunflower . . . the sun is the Communist Party; the sun is Chairman Mao!"

Much of the education in kindergartens during the Cultural Revolution period used examples which instilled a respect for work and an identification with those who do manual labor. In 1971 the teacher during an arithmetic lesson described how the Red Guards, children who have been selected to be members of a quasi-political, extracurricular organization, use their Sundays to help the commune: "They collect four wheelbarrows of nightsoil in the morning to serve the people of the commune and five wheelbarrows of nightsoil in the afternoon to serve the people of the commune. How many wheelbarrows of nightsoil do they collect in all to serve the people of the commune?" During this period writing Chinese characters in one class was taught through copying "Unite to Win Still Greater Victories" from the blackboard. Art class, sometimes called "Revolutionary Art and Culture," often yielded pictures of Tiananmen Square in Peking with brightly colored balloons trailing banners extolling Chairman Mao, crayon drawings of Chairman Mao's birthplace in Shaoshan, or military themes. There were also the occasional pictures of the sun, trees, and birds or a boat or snowman, but these were relatively rare.

During the early 1970s kindergarten children participated in what the Chinese termed "productive labor." They wiped off their tables, washed out their towels, and raised vegetables in the back of the kindergarten. The purpose, according to one of the teachers, was "to better understand the growing process." In one Shanghai kindergarten four- and five-year-olds spent one period a week folding small boxes which were to be used for exporting crayons. In the Gongjiang Kindergarten in Shanghai, in addition to helping to keep the school clean, five- and six-year-olds spent thirty minutes each week folding and stapling boxes into which were packed tiny light bulbs made in the neighborhood factories.

The chasm between manual and intellectual labor had been particularly wide in pre–Liberation China, where Mandarin scholars, with their long robes and fingernails, felt profound contempt toward manual labor. In addition, the rigid examination system formally separated one group from the other, thereby enlarging the gulf between the two. These forms of "productive labor" were therefore designed to serve multiple purposes: they were to provide the children with concrete ways of contributing to their society, they were to enable them to understand through direct personal experience the process of manual labor, and they were an effort to induce respect in young people for the work and the role in society of the worker and the peasant.

"In the last three years, Chinese schools and colleges have been gradually led on to the correct path. Many useful practices common before the Cultural Revolution have been restored and improved," according to a recent article in *Beijing Review*.[23] Over the past few years there has been a fundamental shift in the goals and methods of the Chinese educational system. According to a recent speech by the Minister of Education, "the sabotage to education during the chaotic ten years (1966–1976) was tremendous. The equipment and installation of many schools were wrecked and . . . the losses in manpower were even greater." The Minister continued, "The present state of affairs in education falls far short of needs for the country's modernization."[24]

The educational system is currently being reorganized to support the thrust toward increased production and rapid modernization, to reflect the current Chinese concern with level of knowledge, specific skills, and high general ability. The Chinese educational pendulum, constantly in motion, has swung from an emphasis on political ideology to an emphasis on technical skills or, as the Chinese would say, from "red" to "expert." But as there was a certain emphasis on expertise during the highly politicized period of the Cultural Revolution, so there remains some emphasis on political ideology during this current period. A recent newspaper article discusses the issue of "red" and "expert" and concludes that *both* political awareness and expertise are needed to "meet the requirements of the country's four modernizations."[25]

What indeed are the current goals of the preschool system during this post—Maoist period of the Four Modernizations? How fundamentally has preschool education changed since the Cultural Revolution and the years following it? What values and attitudes are young children being socialized to have? To what extent does public child-rearing follow the political shifts within China, and what are the implications for the well-being of the children? And finally, how have changes in preschool education been manifested in teacher selection and training?

The goal of preschool education today, according to Zhang Shuyi, a member of the Chinese People's National Committee for the Defense of Children, is to "work for the achievement of the Four Modernizations as early as possible" because "children are the successors of our national cause." The director of a kindergarten described the goals of her kindergarten as "fostering the five loves through work and play." The "five loves" are the same as those mentioned in 1972 except for the significant substitution of "science" for the "leader." This substitution serves the dual purpose of emphasizing science as a part of modernization and deemphasizing the role of individual leaders as part of the de-Maoization effort. Illustrating the current importance of the study of science, a recent article in *Beijing Review* describes a "We Love Science" campaign launched throughout China in 1979. The aim of the campaign was "to make every boy and girl realize the importance of science in the nation's efforts to achieve the four modernizations, so that they will set high goals for themselves and study hard for the motherland."[26]

The nursing room of the Shanghai Machine Tool Plant, a factory famous for training workers to be engineers and technicians, was an unusual preschool facility even in 1971. It was more brightly decorated, had significantly more equipment, and had a higher ratio of adults to children than other similar facilities. But in 1980 it virtually glowed with vitality. Brightly colored mobiles and wall designs decorated the rooms, and the nursery had initiated an unusual educational program for even the youngest children. In the 12-to-20-month-old age group, children were learning to identify parts of the body and other objects through large pictures leaning against the wall. Children in this age group were also learning about geometric shapes by matching blocks to identical shapes on a board. In the 20-to-28-month-old group, when the teacher held up large pictures and asked, "What is the little friend doing?" the children as a group shouted out, "He is doing exercises," or "He is watering plants," or "She is getting an injection." These kinds of activities focusing on improving the children's verbal ability, perceptions, and small muscle coordination were not observed in any preschool facility for children of this age group in the early and mid-1970s.

A recent article in a Chinese magazine, *Zhongguo Funü* (*Women in China*), discusses the importance of education from the moment of birth: "When a baby begins to have sensations, he begins to establish a relation with the outside world ... As time passes, these images internalize, help form the child's character and disposition and determine his intelligence as compared with that of other children"[27] The article continues by stressing the importance of early visual and auditory stimulation and finally raises questions about optimum methods for enhancing "a child's knowledge and ability to think" and about differences in levels of intelligence among children. In the words of one teacher in a neighborhood kindergarten in 1980, "Some learn faster than others; some study well; some cannot come up to the mark." This differentiation of innate abilities was not discussed in the early 1970s, when those who "came up to the mark" were barely distinguished from those who did not. Because of the current concern with maximizing children's abilities and with understanding the innate differences among children, the article continues, it is now necessary "to develop a new science of education in China under the name of 'Educational Engineering.'" As part of this current concern with differences in levels of intelligence, Chinese psychologists have been discussing the possibility of adapting Western-type intelligence tests to the Chinese context and incorporating them to a limited degree in their educational process.

The emphasis on formal learning is continued and intensified at the nursery and kindergarten levels. At the Guozi Shi (Fruit Market) Kindergarten in Peking, 240 children who range in age from three to six and one half study five subjects: language and knowledge, counting, music, sports, and drawing. The youngest group of children, who range in age from three to four and one half, have one fifteen-minute class each day; the "middle class," age four and one half to five and one half, and the "senior class," age five and one half to six and one half, have two classes a day, each one thirty-five minutes long. Before the Cultural Revolution, according to the director of the Guozi Shi Kindergarten, there was a teaching program for each class, but during the Cultural Revolution there was "disorder" in kindergartens and the teachers only looked after the children and taught them quotations from Chairman Mao. Now there is a set timetable and they teach prepared lessons which are part of a teaching program organized by the Division of Preschool Education of the Bureau of Education of the Peking Municipality.

A recent article in *Beijing Review* describes a technique used to teach colors to three- and four-year-olds: "The teacher chooses four children in a playground each time and gives them each a different coloured bucket—red, blue, yellow and green. Then she throws twenty small balls painted in those colour on the ground. In this game, the children try to find balls the same colours as his or her bucket, pick them up and put them into their own buckets. The aim is to see who can do it first without any mistakes."[28] It appears at least in this game that learning to compete is a current by-product of learning colors.

Competition, both collective and individual, is being reintroduced into Chinese society at all levels. The importance of competition at the Anshan Iron and Steel Company, the largest iron and steel enterprise in China, has been recently discussed. Formerly, such enterprises felt a "sense of security" because they had a virtual monopoly on their particular area. This sense of security, it is now thought, is responsible for the "current backward state in enterprises." Now that customers can make purchases selectively based on quality, the Anshan Iron and Steel Company has moved from a "sense of security" to a "sense of crisis," a "delightful portent appearing on our country's industrial production scene." For it is only by "putting enterprises in competition to face the world and brave the storm, to compare quality and compete for superiority, will we be able to enable them to catch up with the advanced, become the advanced and bring along industrial development in our country." Consequently, competition among individual workers, among groups within enterprises, and among enterprises is being encouraged.[29]

In preschool settings there is a greater emphasis today than a decade ago on individual activities, particularly on arts and crafts. Drawings are frequently of flowers, a lake, snowmen, or perhaps pandas. Political themes are far less common. The professors at the Shanghai Normal School believe that teachers should encourage students with special interests to spend more time on those subjects and that teachers should also pay special attention to brighter children. There is considerable discussion at this time about the need for more opportunities for young people of all ages to develop their particular talents and interests: "Now it is high time for us to open up outlets for everyone to be free to make progress, for the growth of a generation of talented people along the line of thought of scientific socialism. A series of effective measures should be taken to encourage our people to develop their talents with determination and clear the way for the emergence of new talents."[30]

But perhaps the performances capture most vividly the changes in preschool education. If the early 1970s was the era of such songs as "The Chinese Communist Party and Leninism are leading the cause forward," "We must heighten our vigilance to defend the Motherland," "It is ridiculous to have two Chinas; we are determined to liberate Taiwan!" and, with fierce expressions and fists raised in revolutionary determination, "The poor people of the world must win victories," the early 1980s feature "A dance of welcome for our friends all over the world," "Spring has come; the flowers are all in bloom," a Mongolian milking song, a Tibetan song about picking grain, and "Who can fly? Birds can fly." Perhaps one out of every five songs is one such as the "Dance of the Big Red Flowers," during which four-year-olds sang in 1980 about "obeying discipline, obeying the party, being a good pupil of Chairman Hua and getting a flower" or "Go to see Chairman Hua who overthrew the Gang of Four and kept Chairman Meo's thought in mind for the Four Modernizations in this country," or the ever-popular, then and now, "I love Tiananmen." With the fall from power of Hua Guofeng and the criticism of the "cult of personality," it is likely that there will be even fewer songs praising individual leaders.

Another significant change is the lack of emphasis on productive labor and the corresponding lack of rhetoric about identifying with the workers, peasants, and soldiers. While physical labor remains one of the "five loves," children's participation is limited to washing their own towels and/or smocks, distributing chopsticks, helping to clean the classrooms on rotation, and occasionally watching adults do physical labor. Academic learning has clearly taken priority over participating in work.

But what of mutual aid, mutual caring, the "learning to love each other, help each other and care for each other" that was characteristic of the Cultural Revolution period? According to Gao Zhizhang, Deputy Director of the Shanghai Normal School, "During the heyday of the Gang of Four, children were taught to memorize Chairman Mao's essays without attention being paid to the ability of specific age groups to understand the content. Today the children are encouraged to learn from each other and to help each other but the methods have changed. They are taught not to think of themselves but to see themselves as part of the collective." The Director of the Guozi Shi Kindergarten corroborated this approach: "The children are taught to learn from each other and love each other but not through citing Chairman Mao."

Values and attitudes which were taught under a political banner a decade ago are now being taught under the rubric of "ideological and moral teaching." In March 1981 the Ministry of Education announced that all primary schools (and what primary schools are asked to teach will seep down to preschools in diluted fashion) would introduce "ideological and moral teaching" as part of standard curriculum in the fall of 1981. The Ministry's announcement states that primary schools should emphasize the "lofty ideals of Communism and hard study to realize China's modernization; ardent love for the Communist Party and the socialist motherland; readiness to give wholehearted service to the people . . . ; fondness of labor and the fostering of diligence, honesty, modesty, hard work and plain living; and discipline and respect for the law and public order, concern for public property and pleasure in helping others."[31] It is, of course, no accident that these attitudes are not being couched in political terms but rather in ideological and moral terms. There is considerable evidence that Chinese people of all ages, particularly young people, feel alienated from a more frankly political approach. In March 1980 what was once called "productive labor" was termed "civic consciousness." According to the Xinhua News Agency, "Some 30,000 primary and middle school students gave the capital a treat today in the form of a massive civic consciousness campaign. They turned out to sweep the streets, clean shop windows, help passengers, and publicize hygiene and traffic rules in a 'do a good deed' campaign . . ."[32] As the Chinese have renamed hospitals and roads during and since the Cultural Revolution, so do they appear to be renaming values and attitudes. Much of the desired behavior has not changed, simply the terminology. As in the early 1970s, helping other children is a technique frequently used to deal with very active children. Brighter children are encouraged to help slower children; in one Shanghai kindergarten more advanced and slower children are seated together to facilitate the helping process. Although grades, examination results, and competition are now characteristic of education at higher levels, preschool education continues to encourage mutual aid and cooperation.

The active efforts to foster these values is epitomized by the final pantomime song and dance of a performance at a Shanghai kindergarten. A six-year-old girl dances out "very happy because the people's commune has a bumper harvest this year." She attempts to pull up an enormous turnip but cannot because the turnip is so big. She doesn't "lose heart," however, but calls out to other commune members, all girls, and they too try to dislodge the turnip, but without success. In desperation they form a straight line and, pushing and pulling in concert, they finally dislodge the turnip, singing victoriously, "When we're united, we have greater strength."

Who are the adults who are teaching, guiding, and socializing these children? During the early 1970s some of the teachers were those who had been trained prior to the Cultural Revolution, but the vast majority were either junior middle-school graduates (eight years of schooling), senior middle-school graduates (ten or eleven years of schooling) or "aunties" chosen from among the workers in the factory in which the nursing room or nursery was located. In the rural areas, care-givers were generally older women or young girls who were particularly giving and enjoyed taking care of children. Since teacher training schools and short courses were closed during the late sixties and early seventies, replenishing the supply of trained teachers was virtually impossible.

Today, while there are still substantial numbers of preschool teachers who are junior or senior middle-school graduates with no further training, significant numbers are being trained in short courses designed and administered by the Bureau of Education of the locality to be served or in normal schools. The curriculum for training teachers both in normal schools and in shorter courses emphasizes teaching techniques and the study of child health, child development, and child psychology. In keeping with China's current emphasis on expertise, students who are accepted to normal schools are selected in large part on the basis of their scores on the university entrance examination. In addition to a minimum examination score, professors at the Shanghai Normal School state, the students are expected to have "strong feelings about becoming a teacher, warm feelings toward children and some special ability in the areas of singing, dancing and drawing." The candidates for the Shanghai Normal School, for example, have personal interviews to help the faculty determine their suitability for becoming teachers.

All the students are women, for, again according to leaders of the Shanghai Normal School, "Women are more suitable, more gentle and caring, more able to give motherly love." This emphasis on "motherly love" has been manifested in an emulation campaign to "love the children as their own mothers would."[33] The slogan "loving the children as their own mothers love them" was widely promulgated in 1959 and 1960 but then attacked as "bourgeois theory" during the Cultural Revolution. Now in addition to being encouraged to love the children, teachers are urged to teach them scientifically according to the children's age, mentality, physiological characteristics, and "natural" inclinations.

The Shanghai Normal School, which was closed from 1969 to 1973 because of the Cultural Revolution, currently enrolls 600 senior middle-school graduates in a two-year curriculum. The curriculum includes Marxist-Leninist philosophy, the history of the Chinese Communist Party, teaching methods, children's literature, music, dancing, handicrafts, and science. During their first year the students also take an extensive course in child health, which is taught by a physician and includes human anatomy, nutrition, children's hygiene and health care, the prevention and treatment of common diseases, first aid, and how to measure blood pressure, listen to the heart, and take the pulse. A child psychology course includes material on the "basics of psychological development," on sensations, feelings, memory, attention, thinking, imagination, language, emotion, and personality. In addition, the students study the child's mental development from the ages of three to six. Normal school teaching clearly has not caught up with the current practice, at least in some facilities, of teaching cognitive material as early as one year.

An extremely low level of aggression continues to characterize the behavior of Chinese preschool children. Rarely are children observed hitting, pushing, shouting, taking a toy away from another child, or even crying. According to professors at the Shanghai Normal School, the causes of aggression in children are either hereditary factors, which have only a "slight influence," or the family environment. They do not feel that aggression is "natural" but rather that children are more aggressive when their parents are more aggressive. They attempt to teach their students to analyze the causes of a child's aggression and then to use "positive methods"—organizing special activities for the active child, helping the active child "bring his initiative to other areas," telling stories to educate the child about other modes of behavior, and praising positive behavior—in order to modify the child's behavior. Although the professors are familiar with Freudian and other Western theories of psychology, few if any are included in the curriculum.

At a recent meeting on the "healthy growth" of China's children called by the secretariat of the Central Committee of the Chinese Communist Party and attended by representatives of 31 ministries and organizations, a representative of the Women's Federation advocated the raising of wages and "social status" of nursery and kindergarten teachers.[34] Preschool teachers' salaries do seem to be significantly lower than other workers' salaries. In a Peking neighborhood kindergarten in 1980, for example, the beginning teacher's salary was 35.5 yuan per month and the highest salary was 54 yuan per month. Free laundry and food were provided as well, bringing the highest salary up to the equivalent of just over 63 yuan per month. Beginning factory workers' salaries in state-owned enterprises are approximately 50 yuan per month.

During the past two years there has been considerable activity on the national level around many aspects of the care of children. A National Coordinating Committee on Children and Youngsters' Work has been organized to coordinate nationwide work on preschool education and child care. This committee consists of 16 governmental and mass organizations, with the Women's Federation as the leading agency. In addition, a Cultural and Literary Council for Children has been organized to focus on "spiritual work for children." This group will be concerned with providing books, movies, and other resources. A National Council on Daily Necessities for Children will concern itself with children's clothing, toys, nutrition, study equipment, and other similar issues. One problem the National Council is currently working on is the style of the Chinese school book bag, which has only one strap. Because the students always carry the book bag on the same shoulder, it is said that they develop "uneven shoulders"; the Council is now developing a backpack style of bag with two shoulder straps.

As the political focus has changed dramatically in China over the past decade, the content and teaching techniques within preschool facilities have also changed. In keeping with the current Chinese policy of rapid industrialization and modernization, the preschool system currently reflects the larger society's preoccupation with the acquisition of skills and knowledge rather than the highly political approach of the Cultural Revolution period. There is significantly less emphasis on minimizing class differences through identification with manual laborers and participation in manual labor and increased teaching of concepts and skills early in the preschool sequence. Furthermore, while the group remains the primary focus, individual interests are being encouraged to a far greater extent than during the previous period.

Preschool care in China does, however, still attempt to inculcate feelings of patriotism, nationalism, and commitment to the motherland. It encourages cooperation, mutual aid, a sense of belonging to a collective. The preschool experience encourages the children to view themselves as active participants in a society which they can help to mold; it helps to demystify the workings of that society by encouraging the children to analyze and solve societal problems through song, dance, stories and other activities. And above all, preschool education socializes children from all levels of society to be concerned not only with private goals but to be actively involved in the development of the entire society.

As the small groups of the workplace and the neighborhood help Chinese adults to understand and participate in their society so do the nurseries and kindergartens interpret that society to preschool children and help to socialize them to live within it. The question that remains is whether preschool institutions will move further toward individualism and competition as the larger society moves in that direction or whether they will continue to emphasize cooperation and collective thinking within a society which is moving increasingly toward competitiveness and individual incentives.

7 Education: "Red" versus "Expert"
by Mark Sidel

Educational policy has always been a divisive political and social issue in China. From Confucian times, when arduous examinations were used to select scholar-officials, through the bitter debates over educational "modernization" and "Westernization" during and after the May Fourth Movement of 1919, to the 1980s, when educational reform and educational modernization are once again official policy, differing perspectives and policies in education have mirrored and symbolized wider political and social divisions among China's leaders and within Chinese society.

It was not until 1951, two years after the 1949 Communist victory, that a systematic plan for the reorganization of Chinese education was announced. Premier Zhou Enlai said in 1951 that formal education was to be based on five levels patterned closely after the Soviet system of education. The levels were: (1) preschool education (ages 3 to 7), (2) primary schooling, both for children from ages 7 to 12 and for adults and uneducated youth, (3) four categories of middle schooling—six-year school for 12- to 18-year-olds, schools for workers and peasants, spare-time schools, and vocational middle schools, (4) higher education, including specialized and technical colleges as well as universities, and (5) institutions providing political training for cadres.

From 1951 to 1957, Soviet methods of hierarchical and centralized educational planning were used to guide China's educational system. Russian technicians and advisers streamed into China, while thousands of Chinese students studied in Soviet institutes and univer-

sities. Thousands of Soviet textbooks and teaching guides were translated into Chinese, and Russian quickly became the primary foreign
language taught in Chinese schools.

By 1957, eight years after the Communists had taken power,
impressive gains had been made in Chinese educational work. The
number of students enrolled in primary schools had risen from 24
million to 64 million, while the number of middle-school students
had jumped from one million to over six million. Enrollment in higher
education quadrupled, from 117,000 in 1949 to 441,000 in 1957.

In 1958, dissatisfied with the Soviet model of economic development and China's pace of economic growth, Mao Zedong and some of
his colleagues launched the Great Leap Forward. Aimed at increasing
the participation of ordinary Chinese in national affairs and economic
construction, the Great Leap Forward is perhaps most noted for the
extension and popularization of the agricultural commune system
and for the establishment of numerous small factories and workshops
designed to boost Chinese industry. In education, too, new policies
were the hallmark of the Great Leap Forward. These new policies
took two basic forms. First, the Soviet system of educational planning
and the pedagogical philosophy upon which it was based were criticized
for divorcing classroom study and intellectual activity from actual
Chinese conditions and productive work, and a new movement arose
aimed at combining classroom study with productive labor. Hundreds
of thousands of students and teachers at all levels of the educational
system supplemented their classroom study and teaching by going out
to work on the rural communes, in factories, on construction sites,
and in mines. Thousands of schools set up their own small factories,
thus fulfilling both the call to merge classroom study with manual
labor and China's needs for a higher industrial capacity.

Second, under a policy dubbed "walking on two legs," educational
opportunities were expanded in new and important ways. Communes
and factories were encouraged to open new schools to provide learning opportunities for new groups of students in order to complement
the state schools. In the rural areas, for instance, communes set up
thousands of new primary and middle schools for pupils who had not
been reached by the state-run schools. A particularly good example
of this new policy, as well as of the decision to combine study and

manual labor, was the establishment of thousands of agricultural middle schools of a new type. In such schools students studied for half the day and worked for the other half, thus receiving classroom education while continuing their agricultural work.

During the period of the Great Leap Forward, new policies were developed on an issue which would plague Chinese education for the next twenty years—the proper balance between being "red" (having advanced political commitment and consciousness) and being "expert" (having high-level technical or academic competence). In this period (as opposed to the earlier period of Soviet-style education), the balance shifted to being "red" and to "putting politics in command." Such debates, and the policies of the Great Leap Forward, created considerable controversy in Chinese political and educational circles. The debates—and the changes of policy—over the question of "red versus expert" were to continue until today.

By 1960, the Chinese government recognized that the pace of some of the Great Leap Forward programs (especially in industry) had been too fast, and these economic considerations, combined with rapidly deteriorating relations with the Soviet Union and the ultimate withdrawal of Soviet advisers and cutoff of Russian aid, mandated an important readjustment in many areas of Chinese policy. Educational policy, like economic policy, was affected by these political and economic problems. By 1961 there were new calls for deemphasis of the previous stress on being "red" in educational policy and for a greater stress on technical expertise and classroom study. Classroom periods which had been used for political study and manual labor were returned to the regular academic curriculum so that students and teachers could have more time for traditional classroom work. Some of the schools opened by rural communes and urban factories were closed because of the financial burden they put on those enterprises' resources, and a process of "streamlining," intended to eliminate unnecessary texts, courses, and sometimes even whole schools, took place throughout the educational system.

By late 1963, and continuing in 1964 and 1965, however, new debates over educational policy arose. In large part these debates were a reflection of a continuing and deepening philosophical and political conflict between Mao Zedong and China's President, Liu Shaoqi, who would later fall from power during the Cultural Revolution. During 1964 and 1965, Mao and his allies in the education field criticized the reemphasis on technical expertise, saying that not enough political study was being done and calling for more manual labor in combination with classroom work. Mao and his colleagues criticized the school curriculum, which they said often contained too many courses, and the examination system, which they charged treated students as enemies. They severely criticized the educational system favored by Liu and his associates and adopted in the 1960–1963 period, which closed many of the half-work, half-study schools and set up a two-track system of "key" schools (which were given extra resources and were to serve as national and local model schools) and "regular" schools. Thus, by the beginning of the Cultural Revolution in early 1966, a vigorous debate— with ever-changing policies—was taking place in Chinese education.

Although the opening salvos of the Cultural Revolution were fired in a debate over Chinese culture and drama, the controversies and the struggles over educational policy quickly proved to be not only representative of the political debates on which the Cultural Revolution was based but on the important political conflicts themselves. The Cultural Revolution began in middle schools and universities, and it was from universities and middle schools that the vast majority of China's famous Red Guards were drawn. Chinese educational policy would thus be one of the young Red Guards' primary targets in their criticism of "revisionist" and "bourgeois" policies and institutions.

Soon after the beginning of the Cultural Revolution in 1966, Mao's call for China's young people to struggle against "revisionism, bourgeois ideology, old ideas, old habits, and old culture" took root in the schools. Thousands of students joined the Red Guards, and the schools were formally closed after the summer vacation in 1966 so that the Red Guards could "carry out the Cultural Revolution." Educational policy itself was also transformed, although few schools in which these new policies could be put into effect would be in session from 1966 to 1969. The new policy was to be aimed at "education serving proletarian politics and education being combined with productive labor." In 1966, Mao and others leading the Cultural Revolution again called for a shortening of the curriculum, a reduction in the number of required courses, and a transformation of teaching materials once schools were reopened.

Primary and secondary schools began to reopen in 1968 and 1969, and, as during the Great Leap Forward, many of these newly reopened primary and secondary schools were run at the local levels rather than by state organizations. In addition, thousands of "May Seventh Cadre Schools" were set up in order to give city-based cadres opportunities for manual work in the countryside and political study. While schools had been closed between 1966 and 1969, thousands of young Red Guards received their education "on the streets"—attending political meetings and rallies, reading and writing wall posters, and traveling throughout China to spread the Cultural Revolution. For teachers, the Cultural Revolution was an especially hard period. Thousands were criticized for stressing academic work over political consciousness, and many professors and teachers died during the factional fighting which engulfed China's schools.

Chinese colleges and universities began to open their doors once again in 1970 and 1971, one or two years after the primary and secondary schools. When schools reopened, the curriculum was cut to ten years from the previous twelve for primary and secondary schools and to three years from the previous four- or five-year curriculum for colleges and universities. Political study and manual labor were emphasized. During the early and mid-1970s, this emphasis on political study and manual labor was reduced very gradually, although politics and being "red" remained dominant in educational policy. All students were required to go to work, usually for two years in the countryside, after graduating from middle school. University entrance exams were abolished, and students were admitted to college based on recommendations from Party cadres and their peers.

Periodically, until 1976, China's schools were rocked by political campaigns organized by the Party leadership in Peking. The campaign criticizing Lin Biao and Confucius which took place in 1973 and 1974 is but one example of such political campaigns.

By 1976, the Chinese "revolution in education" had been going on for nearly ten years. Educational policy during the Cultural Revolution represented an extreme expression of one side in the "red versus expert" debate. In October 1976, however, when the Gang of Four, the primary proponents of the "revolution in education," were arrested a month after Mao Zedong's death, "left-wing" policies in education were rapidly phased out. From then on, the pendulum of Chinese educational policy would swing back once again to the "expert" side of the controversy.

Since the death of Mao Zedong, the arrest of the Gang of Four, and the rise of Deng Xiaoping to national power, educational policies and practices in China have undergone dramatic changes. The shifts, discussed in detail in the following pages, may be summarized as follows:

A renewed stress on study and academic performance. Academic study is now considered to be the primary activity in the educational system, and political study and manual labor have been relegated to a secondary role. According to the new Chinese leadership, the new policies on education and toward intellectuals pose no contradiction between being "red" and being "expert." Those in schools, according to Deng Xiaoping, can do their best for China if they work hard to learn or teach as much as possible in their fields of specialization.

A new policy toward intellectuals. The new Chinese leadership has stressed the importance of intellectuals in China's modernization program. The new policy toward intellectuals emphasizes that they should not be sent to the countryside to do manual labor but should be encouraged to work, with as few constraints as possible, in their specialized fields in city-based universities and research institutes.

The return of examinations and competition in schools. Examinations and grades are now given in schools at all levels, from primary school to graduate research institutes, and competition among students is praised as being the best way to motivate both students and teachers and to train the specialists needed for the modernization program.

A raising of academic standards at all levels. At each level beginning with primary school, more advanced academic results are now expected. Toward this end textbooks have been revised or new textbooks written, students and teachers trained during the Cultural Revolution are being retrained, undergraduates and graduate students are being sent abroad, and foreign lecturers are being brought to China in increasing numbers to lecture on the most recent developments in their fields.

The beginnings of restructuring in the educational system. The structure of the educational system is slowly being reformulated with the goal of producing not only highly trained specialists but also middle-level technicians, teachers, and other skilled workers needed for modernization. Primary schooling is being consolidated and lengthened; middle-school education is being lengthened; a new balance is now sought between academic middle schools and vocational middle schools; higher education is being greatly expanded with the focus on science, engineering, and teacher training; and graduate education is being restarted and expanded.

A system of state-emphasized key schools is being established. In order to produce highly trained specialists as quickly as possible, certain schools at the primary, secondary, and university levels are being designated as key schools and will receive special resources from government authorities at the county, city district, municipal, provincial, and national levels. Such schools are intended to be centers of academic achievement, new teaching methodology, and scholarly research. By 1981, there were 96 key universities at the national level administered directly from Peking and thousands of key primary schools and middle schools throughout China.

Enrollment policies are being changed. Beginning in 1977 admission to senior middle schools, technical schools, universities, and graduate schools has been based strictly on results from national entrance examinations rather than on the previous "recommendation" system in which admission decisions were based on political outlook, work results, and the recommendation of fellow workers and Party officials.[1]

Administration

The Ministry of Education is the central government's primary agency for implementing national policy objectives in education. The Ministry's responsibilities include primary, secondary, tertiary, and graduate education; budgets; and teacher training. The Ministry's tasks now also include administration of university entrance examinations and overall supervision of university curriculum. In addition, in 1977 the Ministry was given responsibility for overseeing the preparation of standard textbooks throughout the country.

Below the university level, school systems during the Cultural Revolution had considerably decentralized decision-making powers. In the countryside, for instance, most authority over education policy and work was decentralized from the county education offices to the level of the commune and even the production brigade. Beginning in 1978, this policy was reversed and primary authority for education work in the countryside was returned to the county education bureaus. This newly reinstituted authority includes decision-making powers over enrollment, budgets, teacher and staff assignments, and transfers. County education bureaus also share authority over university entrance examinations and the school curriculum, which remain at least partly under the control of provincial and other higher-level education bureaus.

In smaller and medium-sized cities, basic authority over educational work has once again been returned to the town education bureaus, which hold about the same authority as the county education bureaus. In such major cities as Peking, Shanghai, and Guangzhou (Canton), parallel authority is held by the city district education offices in conjunction with the even higher municipal education bureaus.

Although the great majority of schools are run by county education bureaus, town education bureaus, and city district education offices, there are still some schools at all levels run by other organizations. The greatest number of these are primary and secondary schools run by such organizations as factories, universities, and railroads for children of employees of those institutions. In virtually all *educational* activities (including such areas as curriculum and teacher assignment), these schools are run by the appropriate county, town, or city district education bureau. In *budgetary* matters, however, the factory, university, or other institution is responsible. Generally, these schools have larger budgets because the leadership of the factory, university, or other enterprise is more directly susceptible to the demands of staff members in those organizations for high-quality education for their sons and daughters. While the primary schools run by organizations such as factories and universities are generally open only to the children of their employees, junior and senior middle schools run by these organizations are often open to all eligible students through competitive examinations. Many of these junior and senior middle schools, especially those operated by universities, are also key schools, which are the most important kind of special school.[2]

Key (or "key-point") primary and secondary schools are run by national, provincial, or municipal government departments. They are intended to serve as schools of especially high quality, to produce in the quickest possible time highly trained candidates for college in such areas as science, engineering, and foreign languages. Key primary schools and middle schools may be run solely by education bureaus at the provincial, municipal, or city district level, 'or they may be run jointly by those education bureaus and by other organizations such as universities or other government departments. In 1980, for instance, the city of Peking had three kinds of key primary and middle schools: district key schools, run by the district education office and open by examination to all students living in that city district; municipal key schools, run by the municipal education bureau and open by examination to all students in Peking; and national key schools, generally run jointly by the Peking municipal education bureau and universities and open by examination to all students living in Peking. Among the national key schools in 1980 were, for example, the Peking Foreign Languages School, a division of the college-level Peking Foreign Languages Institute, and the Peking Art School, attached to the Central Art Institute. In 1980, China had a total of 5,200 key middle schools and 7,000 key primary schools with a combined enrollment of over ten million students,[3] but there is continuing debate about the appropriateness of key primary schools.

Primary Education

The provision of universal primary schooling was a consistent goal throughout the 1970s. By 1979 it was reported that 146 million Chinese children, or 94 percent of the children within the primary school age group, were attending primary school. In 1949, by comparison, about 24 million children were in primary school, only 25 percent of the primary school age group. Full primary school enrollment has been achieved throughout urban China, while some gaps still exist in outlying rural areas. Due to demographic trends, especially the large number of children born during the late 1960s, until the family planning campaign was reemphasized in the early 1970s, the number of students enrolled in primary schools seems to be diminishing. One hundred forty-five million primary school students were reported enrolled in 1974, and a peak of 150,000,000 was discussed in 1978.[4] It thus appears that the extraordinary pressure on primary schools during the last ten years, which often resulted in class sizes of 40 or 50 and over, may be beginning to ease (see Table 1).

Table 1
Primary Education

	Number of Schools	Number of Students	Number of Teachers
1949	346,000	24,391,000	836,000
1957	547,300	64,283,000	1,884,000
1965	1,681,900	116,209,000	3,857,000
1976	1,044,300	150,050,000	5,288,000
1979	923,500	146,629,000	5,382,000
1980	917,000	146,270,000	5,499,000

Source: Data for 1949 to 1979, China Encyclopedia Yearbook, 1980, *p. 536; data for 1980,* China Economic Yearbook, 1981, *Section 4, p. 206.*

Chinese primary school students attend school for about eight hours a day, five and a half days per week. The primary school curriculum is a five-year program, and in 1980 the Ministry of Education announced the government's intention to restore a sixth year to the primary school program. Children now enter primary school at about age seven, but because there have been complaints in recent years from parents that age seven is too late to begin primary school, it is expected that many primary schools will accept six-year-olds when a sixth year is added to the curriculum.

During the Cultural Revolution, academic and classroom education was substantially deemphasized. Not only was primary schooling cut back from six years to five, but even in those five years political instruction and manual labor took up a significant number of class hours. Beginning in 1977, these policies were gradually reversed, beginning with the manual work requirement. Required periods of productive labor were shortened, and by 1981 manual work was not usually considered a fundamental part of the curriculum.[5] Classes in politics have continued, although in many schools the number of class hours has been reduced to three to six hours per week. Perhaps even more important, the content of politics classes has changed. During the Cultural Revolution, politics classes focused on Mao's works, contemporary political campaigns, and newspaper articles. Since 1977 politics classes have focused on the history of the Chinese Revolution, the Four Modernizations programs, and increasingly on such topics as ethics, moral development, and study habits.

At the same time, academic standards have been raised in other areas of the curriculum. Chinese primary school students now usually study politics, "everyday knowledge," science, art, physical education, and sometimes a foreign language. Since 1977 textbooks in each of these areas have been revised and upgraded, both at the national level in the Peking-based Ministry of Education and in municipal and provincial education bureaus. Examinations and quizzes are now a regular and important part of primary school life, and in most areas grades are given. In many Chinese primary schools, midterm and semester grades are posted on classroom walls so that students can see who is doing well and who is not, in the hope that those who are not doing well will then try to catch up.

The teaching of foreign languages in primary schools is an example of a policy begun after 1976, which has already been sharply amended, and is in addition an example of the continuing limitations of China's educational resources. In 1977 and 1978, foreign language teaching was started in many urban primary schools. Peking's municipal education bureau established English classes for students in grade three in primary schools on a citywide basis, because it was thought that the earlier primary school students began to study foreign languages, the quicker they would master them. Important problems with this approach soon became apparent. Teachers were not highly enough trained to teach English well, resources were stretched thin, and many students going on to junior middle school found no continuity in the foreign language training. In 1980, as a result of these problems, the Peking municipal education bureau decided to cut back English language instruction drastically in primary schools, except for a few Peking key schools.

In addition to their school activities, many of China's primary school pupils are members of a nationwide organization known as the "Young Pioneers." This group of millions of young people, known as "Little Red Guards" during the Cultural Revolution, was chosen for their achievements in academic subjects as well as their commitment to helping each other. Young Pioneer activities include various kinds of community, school, and cultural programs.

Upon graduation at the age of 12, virtually all primary school students in the city, and many primary school graduates in the countryside, go on to local junior middle schools. Some urban primary school students take an entrance examination in Chinese language and mathematics in their last year for admission to key middle schools, but only a few can be admitted.

Secondary Education

Secondary school enrollment has grown dramatically since 1949, although the gains at this level have not fully matched those of the primary schools. In 1979, over 60 million students were enrolled in different kinds of middle schools, compared with about 1.2 million in 1949. The number of middle schools has increased from 5,200 at the time the Communists took power to a high of 195,000 in 1976,[6] but was reported to have fallen to 121,000 in 1980 because of amalgamation of some schools opened during the Cultural Revolution (see Table 2).

Table 2
Secondary Education

	Number of Schools	*Number of Students*	*Number of Teachers*
1949	5,216	1,268,000	83,000
1957	12,474	7,081,000	293,000
1965	80,993	14,318,000	709,000
1976	194,595	59,055,000	2,809,000
1979	147,266	60,248,000	3,191,000
1980	121,355	55,535,000	3,043,000

Source: Data for 1949 to 1979, China Encyclopedia Yearbook, 1980, *p. 536; data for 1980,* China Economic Yearbook, 1981, *Section 4, p. 206.*

The structure of middle-school education has, like that of primary schooling, begun to change since the end of the Cultural Revolution. Before the Cultural Revolution, China had a six-year middle-school curriculum—three years of junior middle school and three years of senior middle school. During the Cultural Revolution, these six years were cut back to five, as localities stressed expanding senior middle-school enrollment. This five-year program continued after 1976, although Peking's leadership indicated clearly that they preferred a six-year curriculum. Because of limitations on financial resources, available teachers, and building space, little was done to lengthen the middle-school curriculum until 1980 when the Ministry of Education announced a gradual program to extend the nation's senior middle-school program from two to three years beginning in 1981 and 1982.

Prior to the Cultural Revolution, there was a sharply defined "two-track system" of middle schools which included basic academic middle schools preparing students for the university entrance examinations and further academic work, and vocational or technical middle schools, out of which students were expected to go to work as skilled workers, technicians, or teachers. During the Cultural Revolution, this two-track policy, which was closely associated with the former head of state Liu Shaoqi and then Party Secretary-General Deng Xiaoping, was severely criticized for contributing to hierarchical education and furthering social statification. As a result, most of the vocational middle schools were closed or converted into basic academic middle schools. During this period a huge group of teenagers graduated from middle school not only unable to go to college due to a severe shortage of university spaces but without real vocational skills. Since 1976 efforts have been made to modify this situation by restructuring middle-school education to provide a more equal ratio of academic middle schools to vocational middle schools.

Virtually all middle schools are day schools, with classes for about eight hours a day, five and a half days a week, ten months a year. The curriculum in a typical middle school (with some variations according to grade) includes politics, history, geography, a science (physics or chemistry), mathematics, English, and physical education. Class sizes are generally large, ranging from 35 to 55 students, and unlike primary schools, middle-school enrollment reportedly increased through 1979. As in all levels of the educational system today, examinations and quizzes are given regularly, not only to determine standing within each class, but also on a county or districtwide basis to determine competitive levels and judge teaching quality.

After years of neglect (or outright hostile policies) toward many teachers, the quality of teaching and the training and treatment of China's middle-school teachers are now being strongly reemphasized. Wage increases for large numbers of teachers were approved in 1979 and 1980, and major efforts are being made to construct new housing for them. The income and living standards of China's middle-school teachers (as indeed for teachers at all levels) remain low, however. Wages for middle-school teachers now range from 50 yuan to about 90 yuan per month. Unlike many factory workers, middle-school teachers cannot earn monthly bonuses, and most receive only small annual bonuses.

Manual labor for middle school, considered a fundamental component of educational policy during the Cultural Revolution, is now deemphasized. Middle-school students no longer do manual labor each week; in most schools it is limited to a few days or at most one or two weeks per semester.

Some of China's middle-school students (as well as many young workers, peasants, soldiers, and college students) belong to the Communist Youth League, the youth wing of the Chinese Communist Party. Important before the Cultural Revolution but criticized and replaced by the Red Guards after 1966, the League saw a major resurgence in both activities and membership in 1977 and 1978.

League members are supposed to serve as leaders in work and study, in political affairs, and in helping one another. Unlike the primary school Young Pioneers, to which most younger students are admitted, there is real competition to be admitted to the Communist Youth League. Students may join at age fourteen, although many are not judged to have fulfilled the political and social qualifications until they are sixteen or seventeen. In middle schools, new League members are chosen by their class League branch, the group of League members within the class, and approved by school officials. At a later age, League membership can be of significant help in applying to join the Communist Party, which is one of the reasons virtually all middle-school students want to join the League.

During the Cultural Revolution, middle-school graduates were usually sent to the countryside or into factories to work for at least two years before they could return to the cities or apply for college. Today middle-school graduates can enter college immediately after graduation if they pass the entrance examinations. Those who do not pass the examinations usually find jobs in city-based factories or other enterprises, or wait for jobs while living at home. Only a very small proportion still go to the countryside.

Higher Education

Beginning in 1977, the Chinese leadership began a crash program, coordinated and led by the Ministry of Education in Peking, to develop tertiary education. Prior to the Cultural Revolution, China's universities were administered through the Ministry of Higher Education. Direct administration by the central government was restored in 1972 through the creation of a special science and education group functioning under the State Council. Under the 1975 State Constitution, the Ministry of Education (also nonfunctioning since 1965) was reinstated, with its responsibilities now extended to higher education. The Ministry is establishing new colleges, reactivating some which had been closed since 1966, and developing new forms of higher education.

While in 1976, at the close of the Cultural Revolution, there were 392 colleges and universities in China with an estimated enrollment of 565,000 students, by 1980 the number of tertiary institutions had jumped to 675, with a total enrollment of just over a million students[7] (see Table 3). These gains, while impressive, are still not sufficient to satisfy either China's needs for trained personnel or the desire on the part of millions of Chinese students to go on to college.

Table 3
Higher Education

	Number of Schools	Number of Students	Number of Teachers
1949	205	117,000	16,000
1957	229	441,000	70,000
1965	434	674,000	138,000
1976	392	565,000	167,000
1979	633	1,020,000	237,000
1980	675	1,144,000	247,000

Source: Data for 1949 to 1979, China Encyclopedia Yearbook, 1980, *p. 536; data for 1980,* China Economic Yearbook, 1981, *Section 4, p. 205.*

Many of the colleges making up the large increase in the number of higher-level institutions between 1976 and 1980 are colleges being reactivated for the first time since the Cultural Revolution. Among China's 675 colleges and universities, 203 (30 percent) specialize in science and engineering and 172 (25 percent) train primary and middle-school teachers. In addition, there are 32 general or comprehensive universities offering programs in both the natural and social sciences as well as the humanities, 56 agricultural colleges, 109 medical schools specializing in either Western or traditional Chinese medicine, 10 foreign language institutes, 9 institutes for training cadres from among China's minority nationalities and studying ethnology, 7 colleges of political science and law, 37 institutes for sports or the arts, 30 finance and economics colleges, and 10 forestry institutes.

Added to the 675 colleges and universities are thousands of higher-level technical schools scattered throughout China. These technical schools are charged with providing vocational training in such areas as nursing, machine industry, and electronics within a two- to three-year curriculum. As with colleges, students are admitted to technical schools through competitive examinations.

Key Universities. Most of China's higher educational facilities are administered by provinces, by large cities, or directly by the Ministry of Education or other specialized ministries in Peking. Beginning in 1977, the State Council began to designate certain institutions of higher education as key colleges and universities to be administered directly from Peking by the Ministry of Education or other ministries, such as the Ministry of Foreign Affairs, the Ministry of Agriculture, or the Ministry of Health. By 1981, 96 colleges and universities had been designated as key institutions; a list is provided in Appendix F. Key universities receive increased budgets for teaching and research, preference in enrollment of undergraduate and graduate students, preference in faculty assignments, and first right both to send students abroad and to receive foreign lecturers. As with key primary and middle schools, the Chinese leadership has expressed its hope that key universities will produce, in as short a time as possible, highly trained specialists in the academic fields needed for China's modernization program. An analysis of the 96 key universities indicates that the Chinese State Council has placed overwhelming emphasis on training scientists and engineers for China's modernization program. Fully 53 (55 percent) of the key universities are scientific and engineering institutions, although such institutions make up only 30 percent of China's 675 colleges and universities. Teacher training institutions, on the other hand, while they constitute 25 percent of all China's colleges and universities, number only two among China's key colleges and universities. There are 17 key general universities, 6 key medical colleges, 9 key agricultural colleges, 2 key foreign language institutes, and 7 key nationalities, political science, law, sports, and arts institutes.

Administration. Prior to the Cultural Revolution, China's institutions of higher education were run on a dual system of joint administration by older scholars designated as Presidents and Vice-Presidents, and a Communist Party committee composed of Party officials who worked in the university. During the Cultural Revolution, both of these tracks broke down, and eventually revolutionary committees, composed of representatives from many areas of university life as well as the People's Liberation Army and outside Party officials, officials that a dual system of administration be reestablished in China's the early 1970s. By the end of the Cultural Revolution, Party cadres had once again resumed their positions of power in most Chinese colleges and universities.

Although direct Party leadership of colleges and universities continued in most aspects of both academic and political life after the arrest of the Gang of Four in 1976, the new leadership in Peking made clear its commitment to improve not only the social status but also the degree of influence held by intellectuals, especially senior professors who were not long-time Party cadres. Thus by 1979 and 1980 there were growing demands by professors and suggestions by some Party officials that a dual system of administration be reestablished in China's college and universities. In some institutions a dual system of administration, in which professors and other teachers are largely responsible for academic work and Party officials take responsibility for political matters, has indeed been reinstated. Within university departments senior professors are now more influential than Party cadres, and a few university departments have begun to elect department heads.

Admissions. Admission to university has long been a divisive political issue in China. The college entrance examinations, which were the determining factor in admissions before the Cultural Revolution, were severely criticized during the Cultural Revolution and abandoned. When some colleges and universities reopened in the early 1970s, a new procedure for admission of students to college replaced the examination system. Under that "recommendation" system, an applicant, who had to spend at least two years working in the countryside or in a factory after senior middle school, was recommended by colleagues and Party officials at his or her workplace according to political rather than academic criteria. Those who worked the hardest and showed a commitment to "serving the people" were to be admitted.

After the arrest of the Gang of Four, the enrollment procedure was one of the first educational policies in which major shifts were made. In late 1977, the Ministry of Education announced that entrance examinations would once again be the primary factor in determining college admissions. The first set of examinations was held in late 1977, and 278,000 students were admitted for the spring semester of 1978. Each summer since then, examinations have been held for university applicants, and students have been chosen for college according to strict academic criteria. In 1978, 400,000 new students were admitted to college; in 1979, 275,000 candidates were admitted; and in 1980, 285,000 were admitted.

Students who wish to apply to college must choose a general area of specialization—science, liberal arts, or foreign languages—and take the required examinations in that field. In 1980, for instance, applicants in science took exams in physics, chemistry, politics, English (or another foreign language), Chinese, and mathematics. Candidates in liberal arts and foreign languages took exams in history, geography, mathematics, politics, English (or another foreign language), and Chinese. Applicants in different fields were, however, graded differently. For science and liberal arts students, the foreign language examination counted for only 30 points, while for potential specialists in foreign languages the examination was worth a full 100 points. The mathematics examination was worth a full 100 points for applicants in science and liberal arts, but was used "only for reference" for foreign language applicants.

Since 1979 education bureaus in urban areas have been urging candidates from urban schools to apply to teacher training schools and to colleges outside urban areas because of the need for new, fully trained teachers and the severe shortage of urban college spaces. The entrance examinations are graded in each locality, and the Ministry of Education then decides on a mandatory minimum grade for admission to the 96 key universities. Each province, autonomous region, or municipality decides on minimums or grade guidelines for admission to the universities under its jurisdiction. The grades and files of candidates are sent to those universities (in an order of preference indicated earlier by the candidates) at which the candidate is eligible for admission. The key universities are given first preference for selecting candidates and select them in an earlier round; then the regular institutes, colleges, and universities select their students, also from the files provided by county and municipal education bureaus.

Until 1981, the college entrance examinations were the most important factor in determining college admissions. Two factors of less importance were a political check and a medical examination, but candidates were rarely rejected on either of these grounds. High school grades or other activities were not used in the admissions process. In 1980, this practice and other facets of the university enrollment system were criticized by high school teachers and college admissions officers who believed that factors such as grades should be used in the admissions process, and that universities should have more autonomy in the selection process. Beginning in 1981, the Ministry of Education announced that these measures would be put into effect.[8]

Curriculum and Teaching. The length of schooling in China's colleges and universities, cut from four years to three during the Cultural Revolution, has once again been extended to four years in order to ensure that students master more academic material. Some speciality institutions such as medical schools have returned to five-year programs, and a few programs are even longer. Colleges and universities are usually in session five and a half days a week, for ten months a year, from September 1 through the beginning of July.

Students in Chinese colleges and universities take a wide range of courses depending entirely on which school and department they are studying in. Within a department or speciality, most students take the same courses. Until 1979, most colleges and universities had full programs of required courses in each of the four years of college. In 1979 and 1980, however, under pressure from both teachers and students and in the belief that greater student choice of courses would motivate the undergraduates, many colleges and universities reduced the number of required courses in the third and fourth years and offered elective courses within each department. Although a full range of basic courses —politics, Chinese language, usually a foreign language, and basic and advanced courses in the specialty—remain required, Chinese universities are gradually moving toward granting their students more power to choose their own courses. At Fudan University in Shanghai, for instance, students in the history department take required courses in politics, foreign languages, Chinese history, world history, and physical education during their first two years. During their third and fourth years few courses are required, and students may choose from among the offerings in Chinese, Japanese, Russian, Eastern and Western European, African, and North and South American history. In most universities, class sizes generally remain large and the lecture method still predominates. In most college courses, students are tested by written examination rather than through writing research or interpretive papers.

Since 1976 a variety of new academic programs have been begun, both within already established colleges and universities and in new institutions. Among them are many new programs in law, business management, industrial economics, foreign languages, and foreign trade, initiated to train college graduates who can work at the national and provincial levels in fields that are regarded as crucial to modernization.[9]

College and university teachers were among those who were, at times, treated badly during the Cultural Revolution. Since 1977, the Chinese leadership, the Ministry of Education, and local education departments have stressed the crucial role college teachers play in the modernization program and have sought to improve their living standards. Wage increases were approved for college teachers in 1979 and 1980. Construction of teacher and staff housing is now occurring on most Chinese campuses. Even more important, the Chinese leadership has stressed raising the social status and academic levels of China's college teachers. Younger teachers (especially those trained during the Cultural Revolution) are being offered opportunities to upgrade their skills; some college and university faculty members are being offered coveted chances to study abroad; and perhaps most significant, China's system of academic ranks has been restored for the first time since 1965. Today China has a system of academic ranks not unlike the American system. Teachers are classified as Professors, Associate Professors, Lecturers, and Assistant Lecturers, and promotions are based on the decision of their departmental colleagues. There is no tenure system in China because college faculty are likely to remain in the same institution for many years and the number of Professors and Associate Professors remains low in relation to the total number of teachers. At Fudan University in Shanghai, for instance, in a faculty of over 2,000, there are a total of 200 Professors and Associate Professors, and over 850 Lecturers.[10] Promotions are made in a three-step process beginning with discussion among all the members of the department, followed by discussion by a committee of senior professors, and final approval by the University. Senior appointments (at the Professor and Associate Professor levels) must be approved by education officials above and outside Fudan University.

The Chinese system of assigning graduating students to work units has continued since 1976. In many colleges and universities, students are given a list of available job placements and asked to indicate their preferences, but it remains the responsibility of Party officials at colleges and universities to assign graduates to work. This system has come under criticism in the Chinese press because it has been noted that many college graduates are unhappy in their assignments or are doing work which is unrelated to the specialities for which they were trained. Unlike the admissions, administrative, and curricular areas, however, no new system of job assignment has yet been implemented, and thus job assignment remains the strict prerogative of the institutions and Party officials within them.

Tuition and Costs.   In order to eliminate financial impediments to further schooling, major efforts have been made to do away with costs to students at higher-level institutions. Tuition, lodging, books, and medical care have long been free to students in Chinese colleges and universities. Students who were working before they returned to school are paid their regular wages by their employer while they study, even though they will not necessarily return to those jobs upon graduation. Students who are not receiving a salary and who have financial hardships due to low family income are given scholarships by the state.

In 1979, experiments were begun at some colleges and universities to award special scholarships to students who excelled in their academic work. This step marked an important departure from the past because scholarships had previously been based only on financial need. By 1980, some colleges and universities in Peking, Shanghai, and Guangzhou

(Canton), as well as in many provinces, had adopted a merit scholarship system alongside the traditional system based on need, with the goal of further motivating their students to perform well academically.

An even more radical departure from tradition began in 1979–1980. Prior to 1979, Chinese students had not been required to pay tuition. In order to expand enrollment in higher education while easing the heavy financial burden such expansion put on the state, some students were admitted to selected colleges and universities as "self-paying day students." These students live at home and pay twenty-five yuan each semester for tuition, an amount which covers only a small proportion of the real costs of tuition to the state and is not a heavy burden to most of the urban families who supply virtually all of the self-paying day students. In addition, these students must pay for their own transportation, food, and books. In Shanghai, for example, over 3,000 self-paying day students were admitted to colleges and universities in 1980, significantly expanding enrollment in that city.

Graduate Education

For the first time since 1965, graduate education was reestablished in China in 1978. The Chinese leadership, especially Party Vice-Chairman Deng Xiaoping, has stressed the importance of graduate education to the modernization program, and although the number of graduate students still remains small, a rigorous program is now under way.

In China today, graduate students are affiliated with institutions in one of three ways. They may be admitted as graduate students in university departments, and most of the universities which had graduate programs prior to the Cultural Revolution have resumed them today. Thus, for instance, students may be admitted to the graduate programs in physics, chemistry, mathematics, Chinese literature, history, economics, and a wide range of other subjects at Peking University. Second, graduate students may be admitted to the Graduate Academy of the Chinese Academy of Sciences, where they study basic courses in their specialities for one year along with a foreign language and then work as graduate students and researchers in the appropriate research institute under the Academy of Sciences for their final two years. Third, they may be admitted into the Graduate Academy of the Chinese Academy of Social Sciences, where they study in a three-year program which is combined between the Graduate Academy and the appropriate research institute under the Academy; a list of the institutes of the Chinese Academy of Social Sciences is given in Appendix G.

In 1978, the first year in which graduate students were accepted, 10,708 were admitted through competitive examinations to 208 universities and 162 research institutes. In 1979, 8,231 candidates were admitted, 7,646 to universities and research institutes, 261 to the Academy of Sciences, 157 to the Academy of Social Sciences, and 167 to other provincial and municipal organizations. Fewer numbers of students were admitted after 1978 because of the shortage of funds in both the universities and the academies, which has affected undergraduate and graduate education and enrollment.[11]

Admissions

Students are admitted to graduate school based almost exclusively on a battery of five tests given each summer by the Ministry of Education, the Academy of Sciences, the Academy of Social Sciences, and the universities. Two of these examinations, those in politics and a foreign language, are set by the Ministry of Education in Peking. The other examinations, a general examination in the student's field (e.g., history), an examination in the student's speciality (e.g., Chinese history), and an examination in the student's specific area of concentration (e.g., history of modern Chinese-Japanese relations), are set by the universities or the relevant academy. Potential students must be under thirty-five years old, and if they have been working prior to admission their work unit will continue to pay their salary while they are enrolled. Students are usually admitted for three-year programs.

Curriculum and Teaching

Graduate school courses, often led by senior professors, focus almost exclusively on courses in the students' special fields and foreign language classes. Politics is a small and secondary part of the curriculum. Unlike undergraduate education, graduate students are expected to carry out experimental work and write research papers. Such research work is an integral part of the curriculum.

Upon graduation, graduate students most often remain to teach or do research within the universities or the research institutes of the Academy of Sciences or Academy of Social Sciences where they had their training. Because of the lack of highly trained specialists in most fields, university departments or research institutes which train graduate students are usually extremely reluctant to give them up to other institutions. Partially because of the low salaries paid to college teachers and researchers, they can usually afford to keep the graduate students on their paid staffs.

Beginning in 1981, degrees were awarded to some graduate students when they complete their programs of study.[12] Graduate students in three-year programs will generally be awarded master's degrees or Ph.D.'s depending on their performance on their thesis or final project, as well as written and oral degree examinations.

As part of the Chinese leadership's long-term plan to train highly educated specialists, the Chinese Academy of Sciences and the Ministry of Education have cooperated to send hundreds of graduate students, largely in the natural sciences, abroad for training since 1979. Most of these students have gone to the United States, Japan, and Western Europe on government scholarships, and some will earn degrees while they are abroad.[13]

Spare-Time and Adult Education

In addition to primary, secondary, tertiary, and graduate education, China has extensive programs in part-time and adult education for those already working, as well as educational programs for the handicapped.

Since 1976 part-time evening education has expanded rapidly. Many factories, communes, and other enterprises provide part-time instruction, on a voluntary basis, in areas ranging from English to electronics, from art to physics. In 1979, it was reported that over a half-million workers were taking part-time courses in factory-run colleges and spare-time universities, and through passing examinations after such courses workers can be appointed to higher job grades. Another 68 million workers, peasants, and soldiers are enrolled in part-time primary and secondary education.

Yet other avenues for part-time education are courses offered on radio and television. In cities and provinces throughout China, citizens can enroll in a degree program through the Television University. Courses are offered in subjects as varied as English, Japanese, management, electronics, and chemistry. In 1980, a half-million people were reported formally enrolled in the Television University, and many others followed the programs without being enrolled. Courses and exercises are sold in regular bookstores, and homework is assigned on the screen. Many young workers and peasants take part in the Television University or in other such programs, with the hope of upgrading their employment status and moving to more skilled work.[14]

IV | China's and the World's Future

8 | Which Model for Modernization?

In this final chapter we will attempt to discuss the potential impact of China's current modernization efforts on the fabric of that society and, more specifically, on its health and human services. We will then move briefly away from China to examine models of health care in other countries, both rich and poor, and some of the ways in which the Chinese experience has influenced—or failed to influence—these societies. Finally we return to China in an attempt to raise questions about its path for future development.

Modernization After Mao

The China of 1976 was a country buffeted by death, dislocation, and discord: two of its most revered revolutionary leaders had died within nine months of one another. Marshall Zhu De, another revolutionary hero, died in early July; in late July the Tangshan earthquake claimed almost half a million victims, the greatest recorded human toll of an earthquake in the world's history; the Gang of Four, including Mao's widow, were arrested in October just after Mao's death and the obvious question of their relationship to a fifth—Mao himself—hung in the air; Deng Xiaoping was ousted from his leading position in April 1976 but by 1977 was back stronger than ever. It was a society fragmented and demoralized by rapid changes in political ideology, shifts in leadership, and factional disputes. Ten short years before young Red Guards had marched into Peking's Tiananmen Square waving their red books and shouting in one voice, over and over, "Mao Zhuxi Wansui" (Long live Chairman Mao!) but by 1976 Mao, the Chairman, the Helmsman, the symbol of the revolution, was dead and much that he stood for in his later life was coming under severe scrutiny. What were the people of China to believe now? In whom were they to believe? Was it to be Hua Guofeng, a relatively unknown and younger man, identified with Mao's philosophy and with the Cultural Revolution, whose accession to power came about because the aging and obviously ill Mao is alleged to have stated, "With you in charge I am at ease"? Or Deng Xiaoping, who had held important posts before the Cultural Revolution, was identified with Zhou Enlai and the "pragmatists," and who had since 1973 twice been close to the pinnacle of power and twice been removed from power?

After two years of high-level debate, by the spring of 1978 the Chinese had a new slogan, a new rallying point to bring them together, the Four Modernizations. In March of that year Deng Xiaoping, expanding on a call for modernization first made in 1964 and then in 1975 by Zhou Enlai, stated in a speech at the opening ceremony of the National Science Conference: "Our people face the great historic mission of comprehensively modernizing agriculture, industry, national defense and science and technology within this century, making our country a modern powerful socialist state." As the Chinese Communists had in the past "mobilized the mass" to participate in the Great Patriotic Health Campaigns, the Great Leap Forward, and the Great Proletarian Cultural Revolution, so they were attempting yet again to mobilize the people of China to participate in a national agenda.

Deng's call for rapid modernization provided a necessary common goal, a common dream, that could promote cohesion and unity during a period of uncertainty and devisiveness. It also provided the much-needed promise of an easier life for China's millions.

Few would deny the need for economic development in China. As one observer has written, "On the streets of Beijing, men and women trudge along with wooden carts loaded with vegetables. In good weather and bad, bicyclists pull carts heavy with bricks for the housing China so urgently needs. Ubiquitous hand tractors, propelled by 8- or 12-horsepower diesel engines, puff along with carts loaded with commodities of every kind."[1] That an easier life, particularly for China's peasants, is long overdue is beyond dispute. What is open for discussion is the shape, form, and direction China's development will take.

While the Chinese refer to their campaign for the Four Modernizations almost as though the effort at modernization were new to China, the process has, of course, been taking place for at least the past thirty years, and in many spheres, during most of this century. Many of the characteristics of countries undergoing rapid modernization have been characteristic of China since Liberation: migration to the cities (which occurred during the first decade after the revolution and has been largely stemmed since the early 1960s), a significant change in the relative roles of men and women, and a marked improvement in the health status of the people. Other characteristics of modernizing countries have been visible in China to a lesser degree. Countries undergoing modernization generally move toward a consolidation or centralization of decision-making in order to achieve greater control, efficiency, and production. China has, partly out of necessity, partly out of ideology, followed the dual course of consolidating political power in Peking and encouraging decentralization in many sectors of the economy. As part of the process of consolidating power, modernizing countries frequently engage in what has been termed "social mobilization," a transfer of commitment from the community to the society, from local interests to national interests. This process indeed appears to have taken place to a certain extent in China, although the very size of the country, variation among regions, and numbers of dialects, climates, and even styles of cooking encourage regional loyalties, indeed regional chauvinism. On the other hand, nationalism is surely the cement referred to in the Chinese saying, "If we are not as cement, we shall be as sand."

Finally, there are characteristics of developing countries that have been relatively less visible in China over the past 30 years: the development of the cities at the clear expense of the countryside; the rapid development of high technology at the expense of "appropriate" technology; the shift to professionalism at the expense of community-based, indigenous networks and leaders; and the acceptance of "Western" or "scientific" forms at the expense of traditional practices. These changes, which are almost universally seen in developing countries, have been much less visible in China, in part because China's pace of modernization to this point has been gradual—a pace many of China's current leaders feel has been far too gradual—and because of the ongoing debate, some would say struggle, within the leadership about the pathways and forms modernization should take.

The very term "modernization," a relatively recent term in use popularly only since the Second World War, is fundamentally a Western concept. It has in fact been taken by many as synonymous with "Westernization" or "Europeanization," or at least viewed in terms of Western models of development. It is therefore not surprising that the term modernization was not widely used in the standard Chinese political and economic vocabulary until after the death of Mao. Simply promoting the word modernization was a political act on the part of Deng Xiaoping and those currently in power in China. The Maoist concept used to describe the direction China's development should take was rather that of the "uninterrupted revolution."

The concept of the uninterrupted revolution included development through constant struggle, through undermining bureaucratic control and emphasizing local initiative and popular participation, through diminishing the differences between mental and manual labor, between the intellectual and administrator on the one hand and the worker and peasant on the other. The Maoist view included the belief that over a long, difficult period the nature of human beings could be altered so that people would be motivated less and less by self-interest and individualism and more and more by altruism and a concern for the collective, that the way to improve life for one was to improve life for all, that all should rise together, leaving none behind.

The Western view of modernization is predicated on a very different set of assumptions—that "industrialization and technological sophistication require strict organizational hierarchy within which a few lead while the less able, less knowledgeable, and less well paid obey; that modern society is incompatible with a radical egalitarianism and with an increasing integration of man's manual and mental capabilities; that men are largely motivated by self-interest rather than the collective good . . ."[2] This view places a premium on the rationalization of economic processes—efficiency, specialization, the division of labor—and consequently on an unequal system of rewards, particularly between "those who *know* and those who *do*."[3]

The differentiation between "those who *know* and those who *do*" is a particularly difficult problem in China, with its traditional Confucian distinctions between those who worked with their minds and those who worked with their hands. One of the crucial benefits of passing the Imperial examination in prerevolutionary China was the assurance that one would be exempt from a life of often backbreaking labor and that one could then live a life of relative ease, with the respect of family and community. Thus the differentiation introduced once again by the imperatives of high technology could be particularly invidious in a society with a relatively brief history of attempted integration of manual and mental work.

While the unrealistic plans for "modernization by year 2000", which were made immediately following the fall of the Gang of Four, have been "adjusted" to more realistic goals, many aspects of technological development and its possible effects on health and human services give rise to serious concern. Recent developments in China indicate the acceptance by those currently in power of at least some of the underlying assumptions of the Western view of modernization: for example, the emphasis on paying workers according to the amount produced, the stress on material rather than spiritual rewards, and the acceptance that some sectors of the society will inevitably move ahead of other, poorer, less-developed sectors.

We do not mean to suggest that these new emphases portend a foreseeable return to "capitalist" rather than "socialist" economic structures. Indeed, the Chinese take great pains in their current publications to point out the differences between their current policies and their definition of capitalism: the private ownership of the means of production and the exploitation of the workers by the owners. Our question, rather, is whether the new emphases will lead to unintended social consequences.

The changes in education most clearly, perhaps, reflect the shift from the Maoist view of modernization to the current Chinese view: the reestablishment of key schools, grades, and examinations; the choosing of university students solely by their scores on college entrance examinations; the emphasis on expertise rather than on political ideology, on quality rather than on spreading educational resources equitably throughout the population; and, finally, the emphasis on competition which becomes inevitable once the other structural changes have been made.

The dilemma, of course, is clear and real: Can a poor society develop technologically without a scientific, intellectual, and managerial elite leading the way? And once such an elite is developed, is it possible to prevent them from becoming divorced from the vast majority of people, from acting in their self-interest rather than that of poorer, less powerful sectors? This dilemma has been clearly delineated by the economist Paul Sweezy: "Running a post-revolutionary society requires administrators, managers, technicians, experts of various kinds; and, compared to ordinary workers and peasants, the people occupying these positions have higher incomes and dispose over substantial perquisites and power. And regardless of class origin or degree of subjection to the dominance of old ideas, those who enjoy such privileged positions soon develop a vested interest in maintaining them and seek, consciously or unconsciously, to pass them along to their children."[4] There are those who would claim that the development of such an elite is one of the necessary social costs of modernization but that it is a transient social cost, that once China has modernized to a certain level then it will be possible to transform productive relations to deal with the "division between mental and manual labor, the separation of administrative tasks from performance tasks, and the relatively advantaged position of workers over peasants."[5]

There is a serious question, moreover, whether even if a managerial, scientific, and intellectual elite is developed, "modernization" as the Chinese are currently articulating the concept can, in fact, succeed in equitably transforming that vast, overwhelmingly rural country or whether the current campaign will merely succeed in creating greater differences between city and countryside, worker and peasant, and mental and manual laborer. Will the Four Modernizations campaign simply put into place, as it has in so many other third-world countries, a thin layer of industrialization in the major urban centers while poorer rural areas fall farther and farther behind?

Insofar as modernization does take place, it is important to recognize that it unleashes powerful historical forces, forces that few societies thus far have managed to control, harness, or mold to their cultural heritage. It was Mao's belief that the "uninterrupted revolution" might be a way of China modernizing without falling prey to the problems endemic in almost all other societies that have undergone rapid change —disruption of community life, alienation, and anomie.

Since the fall of the Gang of Four in 1976 and the start of the Four Modernizations campaign in 1978, significant changes have indeed taken place within Chinese society. In general, a freer intellectual climate prevails—one that seems to enable many Chinese to speak more freely, to behave more spontaneously than during the previous decade. This new climate has especially favored the intellectuals, the group particularly maligned during the Cultural Revolution: musicians are once again practicing and performing, a variety of theatrical forms are being reestablished, scientists are able to focus on their research and share their results with fellow scientists both inside and outside China, and international exchanges are rapidly developing. Education at all levels is being upgraded, from the first year of preschool care through the newly reestablished doctoral programs, content is being emphasized and evaluated, and intellectual excellence is once again being rewarded.

Economically, both peasants and workers seem to have "profited" during this recent period. Peasants' private plots have in some areas been increased, the responsibility system for individual households is being introduced, and peasants are encouraged to sell their produce in free markets. In certain areas the government has raised the amount it pays to peasants for their produce and, while this has tended to raise food prices for urban workers, many workers have themselves received increases in their salaries, for many the first raise in wages they have received in over a decade. With the current emphasis on light industry, more consumer goods are available to families eager to save and pool their still low salaries in order to purchase bicycles, watches, radios, sewing machines, and the newly available television sets.

Changes are also evident in the areas of health and human services. Local hospitals both on communes and in urban neighborhoods are being upgraded with appropriate medical and health care technology, greater numbers of professional health workers are being trained, and attempts are being made to weed out the relatively small number of technically incompetent barefoot doctors. The reestablishment of Red Cross Societies is creating yet another level of health volunteers, particularly in the urban areas. A massive new family planning effort has been launched throughout the country and a far-reaching law on environmental protection has been promulgated. Increased attention is being paid to the handicapped—the blind, the deaf, the retarded.

With regard to the care of children, there is more emphasis, both at the local and at the national level, on specific aspects of child development. From an increased concern with issues such as nutrition, heights and weights, and the development of motor skills to a concern about the availability of preschool care, the training and status of preschool teachers, and the suitability of toys, books, and other children's equipment, a variety of organizations at different levels of government are singling out children's issues as worthy of special consideration and action.

In short, during the last five years efforts have been made to improve living conditions for many groups within Chinese society. But there also appear to be potential social costs that could significantly alter the fabric of Chinese society. The current stress on individual incentives, for example, raises the question of whether self-interest and personal gain are necessary ingredients for increased productivity. There seems to be little doubt that there were problems in productivity during the Cultural Revolution, but was that due to a reliance on spiritual rather than material rewards or to political discord and factionalism leading to economic disruption? In addition to the question of whether increased individual incentives are necessary for modernization, the question must also be raised whether China's current model of modernization will inevitably lead to increased atomization of society. As production is rationalized for the sake of efficiency, as specialization and the division of labor become characteristic of larger sectors of the economy, will the Chinese inevitably lose the sense of shared norms and values that maintains social cohesion and solidarity? Will they lose some of that sense of collective consciousness and commitment that has made possible the incredible transformation within the brief span of thirty years of a country known as the "sick man of Asia" to one with a "high pitch of collective spirit," a "sense of purpose, of confidence, and dignity," and a "deep sense of mission"?

The Chinese have seemed to see themselves not as individuals first but rather as members of groups first—as members above all of families, and then of workplaces, courtyards, production teams and brigades, and ultimately, of course, as citizens of China. If rewards for individual achievement increase—bonuses for factory workers, larger private plots for peasants, a relatively assured privileged position for those admitted to higher education—is it not inevitable that the Chinese will increasingly relate to their world as individuals whose own personal effort and achievement will make the key difference in their lives? And if the "self" begins to assume primary importance, will citizens of China be willing to submerge their own interests, sacrifice their own desires for the good of the larger society? Will they be willing to limit their children to one because the society as a whole must limit the growth of the population? Will they be willing to work in the rural areas just because they are needed there?

And what of the potential social costs of the current modernization campaign to the Chinese family? As we have seen, the present Chinese family is a three-generational unit in which the members are mutually interdependent. The parents, both of whom generally work full-time, are dependent upon the grandparents to help with child-rearing and housekeeping chores; the grandparents are dependent upon their children both financially and for care and concern when they are old and sick; and the youngest generation is, of course, dependent on both groups. Chinese children have in large part modeled themselves on the adults in their environment. As societies modernize, the world that older people are socialized to live in is so rapidly changed that adult role models often become largely irrelevant to the young. In China over the past 30 years the state and Party have stepped in, in the form of the educational system, neighborhood organizations, and youth groups, to help bridge the gap between the feudal ideology often still held by the older generation and the values and attitudes thought to be desirable in a socialist China. At the same time the elderly have remained a powerful force in the socialization process. If modernization accelerates significantly, will the elderly maintain their role in child-rearing or will peers rather than adults become the most significant reference group as they have in other societies in which rapid change has taken place? Can the Chinese family maintain its current stability?

Can it continue to function as a mutual aid group and provide necessary services to the old, the young, and the middle-aged, or will the family inevitably be undermined by a rapid rate of change?

Chinese children have demonstrated the strong sense of identity and self-assurance commonly associated with the emotional security that comes from being reared in the intimate environment of the immediate family and within stable communities in which mobility is rare and consensus in dealing with children common. As societies change and the family and the community are often undermined, young people frequently feel uncertainty about formerly accepted norms and values; the result is often an upsurge of crime and delinquency. Are the current cynicism about politics among young people and the incidents of petty crime and delinquency in the major cities signs of the undermining of values and norms previously accepted in China?

What will modernization mean to China's neighborhood organization? The Chinese are building 13- and 16-story apartment buildings in Shanghai and in other major cities. There is evidence that high-rise living tends to isolate people from their neighbors and from their communities. Can neighborhood organization that was originally developed for a horizontal courtyard structure be adapted to high-rise apartment buildings and, if not, can the Chinese develop an equally effective form of organization to provide human services and minimize feelings of isolation and alienation seen in cities all over the world?

Will the new emphasis on consumer goods, particularly on individual families owning a television set, promote isolation and undermine that sense of collectivity so essential to the functioning of China's residents' committees and neighborhoods? China's production of television sets has risen dramatically since the late 1960s, from 2,000 in 1968 to 181,000 in 1976 and 2,220,000 sets in 1980. It is not uncommon today for a city family to own its own set. Will the Chinese retreat behind their closed doors to watch the flickering screen as people have over much of the industrialized world?

Will the shift toward professionalism undermine the position of local indigenous leaders? Will the shift of political authority from the neighborhood level to the subdistrict offices mean a loss of control at the local level by the community over its own services? Can lines of communication be maintained which will facilitate both top-down and bottom-up interchange? Or, to put it another way, in a more highly bureaucratized, professionalized urban structure will the residents have mechanisms through which their views, needs, and complaints will be transmitted to those in positions of power?

What will be the effects of such competition on the emotional well-being of China's children? There is already evidence that the system of key schools and highly competitive examinations at various levels of education has begun to create problems for young people. There have been reports of students suffering from depression after having failed one of the examinations, of cheating on college entrance examinations, and of violence among those ineligible to take college entrance examinations because of low grades.

Will China's new education policy of stressing grades and examinations promote competition instead of cooperation in the classroom and, if so, at what age will competition dominate children's relations with one another?

Will the current educational policy so favor urban children of professionals and of Communist Party officials that China will once again develop a scholarly elite divorced from manual labor and from the vast majority of workers and peasants? If, as it currently appears, more urban students are being accepted into universities and technical schools because they are better prepared than their rural counterparts, who will serve the 85 percent of the population who live in the rural areas? Will the gap in services between the urban and rural areas grow even wider? If teachers, nurses, and physicians are not recruited from rural areas, who will serve the needs of the immense rural population? Few, if any, societies have been successful in persuading urban dwellers to move to rural areas. Will the Chinese be able to persuade urban professionals to work in rural areas and, if they do, will urban professionals be able to relate to rural residents, rural problems, and rural living conditions?

What will modernization, particularly the changes in education, mean to Chinese women? Since 1949, Chinese women have made great strides despite the long history of cruel oppression they lived under before the revolution. Educational and occupational opportunities were made available on a scale unmatched by any comparable society. Nevertheless, women are far from genuine equality—in the family, on the job, and, above all, at the higher levels of government. If students are selected for higher education solely on the basis of examination scores, will women be equally represented? Will they be sufficiently represented in fields traditionally dominated by men if they are not explicitly sought out and encouraged to enter these fields? In their attempt to train the "best-qualified" people, will the Chinese neglect their commitment to women? In an era in which modernization has priority, will women be given the opportunity to "hold up half the sky"?

And, finally, what will rapid modernization mean for health care in China? The Minister of Public Health, Qian Xinzhong, at a national health conference attended by the leaders of the health bureaus of China's provinces and regions in January 1981, stated their "major tasks" for the year. It was announced that China would "increase its medical expenditures in 1981 as part of the national economy readjustment program which gives a bigger proportion to culture, education and science." The specific tasks included

—strengthening county hospitals and, starting with one-third of them, building them into "standardized medical centers"
—developing the rural cooperative medical service based on the brigades' economic conditions and supplemented by small peasant contributions
—training the "more than 1.5 million barefoot doctors" in a "well-planned way," granting the qualified ones "certificates for medical practice" and reserving a percentage of medical college enrollment for the promising ones among them
—focusing research on "subjects most vital to the health of the population"
—simultaneously developing Chinese traditional medicine, Western medicine, and a combination of these two schools
—family planning
—developing health protection programs that will concentrate on "industrial hygiene, environmental hygiene, the food industry, schools and biologic causes"[6]

In short, based on our own observations in 1980 and on the published official goals of the Ministry of Public Health, it appears that the two "newborn things" of the Cultural Revolution in rural health care—the barefoot doctors and the cooperative medical services—will be preserved and strengthened. There was also evidence in 1980 that the lane organizations for health work—with their Red Medical Workers, now called Red Cross Medical Workers but not substantially changed in function—would be preserved. For the most part the Chinese had managed, at least until late in the decade, to introduce the new technology into an existing social organization at the most local level, rather than changing the social structure to fit the new technology. An emphasis on prevention and on close contact of health services with people had, at least till then, been maintained.

As to the future of health care, there is danger that the drive for rapid modernization may have negative—and perhaps unintended—consequences. Rapid economic modernization may, as Robert Blendon has pointed out, result in a slowdown in the unfinished agenda for rural areas and widen rural-urban gaps in medical care.[7] The "raising of standards" and the increased "professionalization" may lead to less assignment of urban medical workers to the countryside, to the building of larger, more technological regional hospitals in preference to more decentralized primary and secondary care facilities, and to reduction in local management of health care facilities. The general trend toward clinical specialization is likely to increase the wage differentials among professionals and lead to their greater emphasis on treatment rather than prevention. The training of personnel in other countries is likely to lead to wider gaps in their ability to deal with poor people in their own society, to concern with high-technology care or with basic research rather than its applications, and to the demand for even greater centralization of resources.

Moreover, what will increasing introduction of high technology and professionalization do to popular participation in health care? The principle that "health work should be combined with mass movements" has been one of the four cardinal tenets of health work in China since 1959, with precedents going back to the Jiangxi Soviet of 1927, the Long March, and the base at Yan'an. There is little doubt that many of China's awe-inspiring accomplishments in public health over the past three decades have been based on motivating large groups of people themselves to change their environmental conditions to promote health and prevent disease. There is equally little doubt that a high-technology-based, professionalized health care system will have greater difficulty in turning the power to change their own conditions over to large groups of nontechnically trained people. It is of course true that the patterns of disease have changed in China, that infectious diseases are rapidly declining as its major causes of disability and death, and that new forms of environmental protection—concerned less with micro-biological contamination than with chemical waste products and with other carcinogens and mutagens—will be needed. But will technicians and professionals be able to take the place of the "mass" in a country of one billion? And even if, for certain programs, technicians can perform aspects of the work better than the people themselves, what are the consequences for the mobilization of the Chinese people in areas in which mass mobilization rather than technical proficiency is still required?

Another dilemma for China as it seeks rapid technological development in the final twenty years of the twentieth century is whether and how much to borrow from technologically developed countries, both in terms of the technology itself and of the foreign exchange to pay for it. Taking too little means, of course, laborious "reinvention" of the technology, long delays in tooling-up to produce equipment immediately—and often, in the short run, much less expensively—available in the rich countries, and consequent long delays in acquiring the benefits of the technology—whether for improvement in the daily life of people or for defense against national disasters or foreign enemies. Taking too much technology, on the other hand, poses other problems: dependence on other countries, which may "pull the rug out"—as the Soviet Union is said to have done to China in the early 1960s—if the dependent country does not remain a client state; loss of traditional national values, which may be devalued or shunted aside as the imported technology rapidly takes hold or as technical personnel learning in other countries return; and shifts in priorities that are more related to the importation of technology than to national needs. Almost no one argues for an all-or-none position: that a nation must be entirely "self-reliant" or that it should be entirely dependent on foreign technology. The issue, rather, is where to draw the line, how to strike a balance between independence and dependence, and how to improve the material lives of its people without destroying elements that make those lives worthwhile.

In addition to China's new willingness to import large amounts of technology and equipment, it has recently begun to accept foreign aid and to discontinue part of its own foreign aid. As an example of its previous policy of "self-reliance," China had, as discussed earlier, withheld for years the number of casualties (now estimated as 242,000 dead and 164,000 seriously injured) in the 1976 earthquake that leveled the mining center of Tangshan and severely damaged Tianjin and Peking. In contrast, an earthquake in a rural area of Sichuan Province in January 1981—which resulted in relatively few injuries and relatively minor damage—was promptly reported and emergency relief aid from other countries was accepted. This aid included cash and blankets contributed through Red Cross Societies in 14 countries. Over the past two years China has accepted United Nations funds to help it deal with 250,000 refugees from Vietnam and used the United Nations World Food Program for emergency grain and edible oils. The United Nations plans to spend $200 million for development and population control projects in China over the next few years.[8]

In the fall of 1980 China made its first appeal since Liberation in 1949 for international relief aid for people in provinces with severe food shortages due to what have been called the worst droughts and floods in almost twenty-five years. In February 1981 a United Nations team and other international relief officials surveyed the areas and recommended urgent relief aid for the hungry and homeless, reportedly 130 million people facing varying degrees of food shortages in at least nine provinces. The international officials noted also, as reported in the *New York Times*, that "people are not starving and that the government's own relief effort is well underway and seems fairly well organized."[9]

In addition to being willing to accept foreign aid, China has over this same period sharply curtailed its own foreign aid projects. China still makes gestures of aid to other countries—such as its pledge of a modest $1 million in April 1981 to the international relief effort for African refugees. But the days of China's contribution of the Tanzam Railroad in Tanzania and Zambia and of major medical aid to other countries poorer than China are apparently over for the foreseeable future. Chinese officials emphasize that in the past China has always honored its obligations to international agencies such as the United Nations but had "waived its right to benefit." Now China views its participation as a "two-way street" and as a "question of mutual help." The officials declared that self-reliance continues to be a basic principle in China, that the international aid China was seeking was small compared with China's needs, and that the domestic relief effort "far exceeds" donations from other countries.

In its industrialization efforts, China is also seeking the help of international agencies. The government is soliciting low-interest loans from the World Bank, the International Monetary Fund (which approved a $550 million loan in February 1981), and foreign governments and corporations. It has offered, for example, to continue joint ventures with Japan in heavy industrial development—which China had formally canceled—if Japan offers inexpensive loans for their completion and investment funds for their operation. China has, however, apparently remained fiscally prudent so far, refusing loans with high interest rates, unlike other third world countries that have borrowed their way into severe interest-payment problems.

China's official position is that its introduction of foreign technology and equipment will not induce dependence but will "boost our ability to stand on our own feet." Official statements point to low productivity in China, from agriculture, where the average annual grain output produced by a peasant is about one ton, only a fraction of that produced by a farm worker using machines in technologically developed countries, to iron and steel industries. They point to Japan, where they say judicious importation of foreign technology permitted major improvements in productivity without inappropriate dependence on foreigners. They even quote Chairman Mao, who urged China to "make foreign things serve China."[10] But the nagging question of the impact of the foreign technology on China's social organization, on its priorities, and even on its long-term goals remains.

Models for Other Countries

It is ironic that at the same time China is seeking to learn techniques of modernization from other countries, many people of these countries—both technologically developed and developing—are questioning the methods their societies are using and the changes in quality of life that have been produced.[11] Many of those questioning the direction that their own societies are taking have—as we discussed in the introduction—looked to China for possible ways to change what they perceive as dysfunctional policies. Health services are excellent examples of an area in which, as China is increasingly attempting to learn highly technological and professionalized methods from other countries, these methods are undergoing increasing questioning at home. There is no doubt that there have been great improvements in health over the past century in technologically developed countries. But much of this change can be attributed to improvement in nutrition and to the provision of pure water supplies, safe sewage disposal, and, although somewhat more controversial, many forms of immunization.

At the same time as these remarkable advances have been made in the protection of health there have indeed been great strides in the treatment of illness. The introduction of hormones like insulin and steroids; of antimicrobials such as the sulfonamides, penicillin, streptomycin, and isoniazid; of psychoactive drugs such as chlorpromazine; of modern methods of surgery and anesthesia; and of life-sustaining techniques such as hemodialysis—despite the new problems they have introduced—has saved many lives and improved the quality of many more.

Until a few years ago it was widely accepted that the obvious improvements in health in many countries were the result of technical or professional interventions in either the protection of health or the treatment of disease. If a health problem existed, it came to be felt, what was needed—either by the community or by an individual—was the right professional who would introduce the right technological solution that would protect the victims from illness or heal them after they became sick.

Within the past decade, however, a number of criticisms of this model—that of the health "professional" who is responsible for "helping the victim"—have appeared. On the one hand, critics have pointed out that the standard "professional" medical and health models haven't seemed to be of much use so far for what have become the leading causes of death in technologically developed countries: heart disease, cancer, stroke, and accidents. Nor have the professional strategies—

whether in prevention or treatment—been of much use for other major causes of disability and despair in these countries, such as arthritis and other musculoskeletal disorders, mental illness, or abuse of alcohol or other drugs.

Even more disturbing, some critics have questioned the usefulness of the professional intervention model even where it was assumed to have been most useful, in the prevention and treatment of infectious diseases. These critics suggest that it was first the general rise in the standard of living in the industrialized countries—the improvement in food, shelter, clothing, and other living conditions—and only secondarily public health techniques such as pure water and safe sewage disposal that led to the dramatic fall in death rates over the past century, and that most of the professional medical care techniques had little to do with the improvement in life expectancy. While this view flies in the face of the conventional wisdom and has indeed been challenged by some analysts, there certainly appears to be substantial evidence behind it with regard to at least death rates.[12]

Concurrent with the spread of criticisms of the efficacy of medical care has come concern about the enormous rise in its cost. As the percent of older people in the population of technologically developed countries rises and those with chronic illness need and demand care, as the complexity of medical techniques—such as CT scanners and modern surgery—increases, as the number of highly trained people engaged in professional medical care rises sharply, so does the cost of medical care to the society. In the United States the consumer price index for medical care has risen 60 percent over the past five years, more than any of its other components, and the health sector now consumes close to 10 percent of our gross national product, over $1,000 annually per person. The use of this vast amount of money is skewed, with fifty cents out of every dollar going to hospital and nursing home care and less than five cents of each dollar spent on health protection or promotion. Moreover, this enormous burden is unequally distributed and falls most heavily on the poor.[13]

Perhaps most disturbing of all, however, are the criticisms coming from the poorest countries of the world, where even the basic public health measures of pure water supply, safe sewage disposal, and immunization have yet to reach more than a relatively few favored individuals and where infant mortality rates, life expectancies, and access to medical care for illness remain far worse than in the rich countries. Many poor countries spend less than $2 annually per person on health. The setting up, usually with outside help, of "centers of excellence," typically in the cities, or the training of highly professionalized personnel, has had little general impact. Indeed, many of the poor countries suspect that most of the professional interventions donated from the rich countries, even the clearly useful ones like smallpox vaccination or contraception techniques, are designed more to protect people living in the donor countries than to help those living in the poor ones. And even where the giving appears to be truly altruistic, or the changes are made using internal resources, professional interventions often seem painfully slow or ineffective.

In short, in both the poor countries and the rich ones, the "professional" or "help-the-victim" strategy has been increasingly seen as severely flawed.

New models have been advocated to replace this strategy in poor and in rich countries. While these models are quite different from one another, they share a tragic flaw: they can both lead to a net reduction, at least in the short run, in services for those who need them most.

In many of the poor countries, the goal has become general economic development or "modernization." Only general development, it is argued, can bring the improvement in living conditions that will help prevent illness and promote health. While the theory is an attractive one, recently industrializing societies—Mexico and Brazil are good examples in our hemisphere—have for the most part relied on "trickledown" to reach the vast majority of the desperately poor. Income distribution has changed little if at all; the pie is indeed larger, but the poor still see very little of it, and their health status remains extremely low compared to that of the relatively well-off in their societies.

The conditions found in underdeveloped countries are in some measure shared by areas in the United States. Although the United States ranks relatively high in health status among the nations of the world—though not as high as its relative wealth should enable it to do—health and health services are grossly maldistributed.

Health problems of the poor and of racial minorities are much worse than those of the affluent and of whites. Although overall U.S.

mortality rates are declining, the overall mortality of racial minorities is still one-third greater than that of whites, and higher rates are also found among the poor and uneducated. Death rates in every year of life are higher for poor children and highest for poor black children. Infants of racial minorities have almost twice the infant mortality rates of white infants. Life expectancy at birth for members of racial minorities is over five years shorter than that of whites. Nonwhites have three times the maternal mortality of whites, and this difference has not been reduced significantly in the past 25 years. From 1950 to 1975 the age-adjusted cancer death rate for the white U.S. population increased 4 percent; for nonwhites the increase was 20 percent. In a low-income Chicano community in Los Angeles, children were found to have four times as much amoebic dysentery as the national average, twice as much measles, mumps, and tuberculosis, and 1.4 times as much hepatitis.[14]

The Borough of the Bronx in New York City is a particularly dramatic and tragic example of deteriorating conditions in American inner cities. Over a four-mile distance from the North Bronx to the South Bronx, there is an extraordinary increase in visible poverty. In the South Bronx the median income is less than half that in the North Bronx. In 1970 the reported incidence of tuberculosis was six times as high in the South as in the North, of gonorrhea ten times as high, of measles 15 times as high, and of lead poisoning 30 times as high. Infant mortality rates in the South were almost double that of the North, and deaths attributed to drug dependence were almost 25 times as high.[15] In 1970–1972 infant mortality rates in the South Bronx were 19 percent higher than the rate for New York City as a whole; by 1977–1979 the South Bronx rate was 33 percent higher than for the city as a whole. And other statistics are just as appalling.

Health services for the poor and for racial minorities, most of which must be publicly funded, are much less adequate than those for the affluent and for whites. Resources for public health services and for municipal hospitals are grossly inadequate to meet health needs in many cities. Funds for these programs, in real terms, are diminishing in many areas. Public hospitals have recently been closed in Philadelphia, St. Louis, and New York City and are in serious trouble in other cities such as Chicago and Atlanta.[16] Public health departments are being decimated in many cities, including New York, which once had one of the finest health departments in the world.

In short, in the South Bronx and in other poor urban areas of the U.S.—the areas with the greatest health needs—health care and medical care services are actually being reduced through disappearance or irrelevance of private services and budget reductions for public services. These areas share many of the characteristics of developing countries, and dependence on national economic development—or on "increased productivity"—to provide better services and better health for the disadvantaged seems equally unlikely to succeed in the technologically developed countries.

In the rich countries, indeed, a quite different type of strategy from the general development model has emerged—a focusing on the life-styles of individuals as one of the major causes of poor health. The smoker is blamed for his lung cancer, the alcoholic for his liver disease, the driver for his automobile accident, and the hypertensive for his stroke. Like the general development model of many of the poor countries, this "blaming the victim" or "individual responsibility" model in the rich ones is probably a needed correction to total dependence on a "professional" model, but it seems to be equally flawed. Many if not most of the criticized habits and life-styles are culturally or economically determined, and many of the current causes of ill health—such as environmental or occupational illness—are beyond the control of any single individual or family. Life-styles, insofar as they are not genetically determined, are environmentally induced through advertising or peer pressure. In short, some techniques of "mobilizing the mass" already exist in technologically developed countries, but many of these techniques are used to promote consumption, much of it deleterious to health. The question in these countries is how to ensure that the techniques are used to promote health. Another problem with "blaming the victim" is that it at times appears to be simply a method of drawing attention away from societal causes of illness and of justifying the withholding of social resources from the prevention or care of illness.

Where, then, does that leave the concerned people in most of the world's countries? If the professional model, though certainly useful in certain areas, is flawed and inadequate to meet current needs and if its replacements—general economic development in the poor countries and emphasis on the individual in the rich ones—while surely expressing important elements of promotion of health, are equally flawed and inadequate to meet current needs, what model will replace or complement them?

In several developing countries over the past few years models have arisen which may be called the "organizing" or "community" strategies. At root, this model views people as having been culturally and economically forced into positions of underdevelopment, weakness, and high risk. This is true of entire societies, such as the colonial nations of Africa, as well as of parts of societies, such as the inner cities and the Appalachian region of the United States. The answer to underdevelopment, and to correction of unhealthy conditions, is seen as collective action. Only by assuming power over their own lives and over their own environments, and by wielding that power to make substantial change, can people make decisive improvements in their own health.[17]

The country that has been the clearest example of the "organizing" or "community" model is, of course, China. China's demonstration of a poor country's ability to reorganize fundamentally its health care and medical care systems and to produce almost incredible change in the health of its people has been an inspiration to many in poor countries and the poor parts of rich ones.

The direct transfer of China's health and human service models to other countries—whether rich or poor—is, however, almost impossible without the transfer of China's social, economic, and political organization and even its cultural traditions. Indeed, it has repeatedly been pointed out that to view China's health services and other human services as a series of techniques that might be transferable without the social, economic, and political structure that made them possible is to miss the central point of China's developmental experience.[18] Beyond that, it is clear that health and educational services, for example, are only single elements in development—and perhaps not the most important ones—that lead to better health or to better education. It may be possible, nonetheless, for other countries to learn from the principles that China has tried to apply and perhaps to attempt to transfer specific limited techniques. These attempts may stimulate further developmental change in other areas or may, by their very failure, raise the consciousness of people about the structural changes in society that are needed for their success.

There are many examples of health programs that appear to have been directly derived from Chinese models, to have been influenced by China's experience, or at least to have arisen, based on similar needs and similar principles, at about the same time. One such program, mentioned in our Introduction, was an explicit attempt to introduce the "Chinese barefoot doctor" model into rural Iran. This experiment, with new personnel called "village health workers," was only partially successful because of the social, economic, and cultural differences between rural Iran and rural China. The health workers were chosen by the village headman (usually the son or brother of the headman or the headman himself) rather than by the people of the village. It was rare to have a woman selected because of cultural barriers to women leaving the village for training; the preventive and educational aspects of the work (as contrasted with treatment) elicited little enthusiasm; and factional disputes in the villages made selection of the health workers and their work difficult if not impossible. The conclusion: "We believe that the Chinese barefoot doctor is not easily transportable to Iranian soil." [19]

A much more successful example of the development of a health worker similar to the barefoot doctor was seen in Tanzania, one of the world's poorest countries. As part of a social revolution under President Julius K. Nyerere, with the aim of "socialism and self-reliance," there were developed "Ujamaa [which means "familyhood" in Swahili] villages," rural developments whose members join in communal farming and social improvements on a basis of "love, sharing and work." It was not surprising that these villages supported "village medical helpers," selected by fellow villagers, trained at a district hospital for three to six months following primary school education, and concerned with prevention of illness and treatment of common diseases. [20] Similar programs were developed in a number of African, Latin American, and Asian countries.

Yet another example, in a more technologically developed country, was seen in Chile under President Salvador Allende (himself a physician) from his election as a socialist in 1970 to his death in a military coup in 1973. During this period urban medical centers were placed under the control of committees that included strong representation by local residents, and rural assistants were trained to work simultaneously in agricultural development and health care. These programs were immediately dismantled after the coup, and many of those participating in them executed, imprisoned, or exiled as dangerous subversives.[21]

International agencies spread the word of the successful experiments, in China and in other countries, around the world. Books and articles emanating from the World Health Organization appeared under such titles as "Health by the People," "Alternative Approaches to Meeting Basic Health Needs in Developing Countries," "Health Care Development as an Agent of Change," "Health for All by the Year 2000," and even "Bringing Down the Medical Empire" by the World Health Organization's Director-General, Halfdan Mahler, who argued that "before it can truly help improve health conditions, the medical profession must first replace its imperial trappings with a real concern for people."[22]

The Chinese experience in integrating their traditional medicine with Western medicine has also provided a number of lessons for other countries over the past ten years. In developing countries it has encouraged exploration of similar integration of traditional medical care systems with the limited amount of scientific medicine available. As noted in the Introduction, the World Health Organization and other international agencies have encouraged poor nations to use their traditional medicine as an important aspect of the provision of health services. These efforts have included the education of traditional practitioners—such as indigenous midwives—in modern practices and on criteria for referral for more technological help and the introduction of techniques of traditional medicine—such as herbs or acupuncture— into modern practice. One of the problems with traditional medicine in many societies, however, is that it is fragmented into many different systems, often based on magic and witchcraft, and therefore does not lend itself to codification, standard-setting, or integration with "organized" systems of care.

Transfer of China's techniques of encouraging family planning may be even more difficult than transfer of its health care methods. The unprecedented success of the population limitation program in China is clearly dependent on China's intricate neighborhood and commune organization, its group pressures, its nationalism, its methods of rewarding (and of not rewarding) people, and—most important of all—on its people's conviction that they will not be left destitute or alone in their old age if they have no surviving children and that any national gains in standard of living that their sacrifice helps produce will be equitably shared. Countries that cannot offer such organization, group cohesion, and believable assurances—which includes almost all countries in the world with high growth rates—will be unable to emulate China's total family planning program until the other social changes are made. In the short run, the use of specific techniques similar to those used in China, such as the low-dose pill, the experimental morning-after pill, the pill for men, and the use of indigenous workers trusted by their neighbors, may be useful. In the long run, only profound structural change in social and economic organization—or an extraordinary rise in standard of living, undreamed of in most poor countries—will permit reduction of growth rates to the level that China, a relatively poor country, has already attained.

To turn to an example from a technologically developed country, attempts have been made to use some of the lessons learned from China in the North Bronx. In the neighborhood that surrounds Montefiore Hospital, its Department of Social Medicine has sponsored a Community Health Participation Program. The objectives of this program are to develop a community-based network which will encourage people to be concerned with their own health and that of their neighbors on a building-by-building and community basis. Within each apartment building, interested residents are trained as "health coordinators." Health coordinators are not trained as paramedics or as physician extenders but instead serve a very different role, as unpaid "health promotors" for their buildings.

During the past two years, trained health coordinators initiated a number of projects in their apartment buildings, including counseling individual tenants and families on matters of physical and mental health, referring neighbors to social agencies and community help when needed, helping neighbors with particular ongoing health problems (including taking blood pressure of persons requesting it), giving first aid in emergencies, encouraging people to see a doctor when appropriate and accompanying them to the doctor or hospital if needed, organizing cooperative buying, advising neighbors on general health topics, informing tenants of programs and legislation affecting them directly, and organizing self-help groups and health workshops in a variety of areas ranging from stopping smoking to parenting.

The training is actually conducted, whenever possible, at a site which is physically removed from the hospital itself. Because of this physical separation, community residents interested in participating don't view the program as simply another extension of the hospital bureaucracy but as something separate and distinct, with a character all its own, smaller and more human-scaled than the hospital.

On the other hand, the program's affiliation with the hospital has permitted it to draw upon the hospital's resources for specific assistance when needed. For example, each health coordinator has been assigned to a hospital staff member whom the coordinator can contact if a particular health problem is beyond the coordinator's expertise.

Clearly, the health role of the health coordinators in the program is defined broadly so as to include all aspects of neighbors' health. Health coordinators routinely follow up on their neighbors' visits to doctors and on their contacts with social service agencies to ensure that they are receiving adequate services. Coordinators also serve as advocates for services needed by their neighbors and participate in decisions about health care.

Volunteers for the program are recruited in a variety of ways—through existing neighborhood and tenant networks, block patrols, community organizations, individual contacts of other health co-ordinators, and through open workshops on health topics held for the public in the neighborhood.

In the basic training program, health coordinators learn about a broad spectrum of health-related topics: concepts of health, first aid, nutrition, relaxation and exercise, choosing and using a doctor, making the health care system work for you and others, interpersonal commun-ications, community organizing, chronic diseases, the physical exam, addictions, child health, and sex and family planning. Other more specialized training is provided when called for; unlike many other training programs, the health coordinator training is not rigidly planned by the program staff. Volunteers in the program are asked what they would like to learn about health and related matters. And, although certain basic components are always included, the training program is, in large part, designed by its participants.

In doing this work, a number of principles emerge—based in part on lessons from China. First, we as professionals must do nothing that will increase the powerlessness or the dependency of individuals or of the community. Second, stating the point in a positive way, in our work in the community we must whenever possible help to strengthen the determination, channel the alienation and despair, and build the social structures which will permit people and communities to take their destiny into their own hands. This includes fighting alongside them for retention of their publicly supported services. One of the most important ways in which we can do this is to help transfer knowledge and skills into the hands of the community. Third, we must recognize, as we do this, that one of our most important tasks is not as teachers, but as students, learning from the communities their needs and their strengths and learning with them how to produce effective social change and effective health care. The community must become the reference group, the setter of standards. The "diffusion of excellence" must take place from the bottom up rather than from the top down, from the community to the professional rather than in the other direction. As we attempt to build new forms of health and human services in our own society—and to defend existing forms against attack—we would do well to learn from China's successes and from China's failures.

Models for the Future

Returning to China, while its vast accomplishments of the past 30 years can serve as models or as inspiration for other countries, there remain large urban-rural gaps in income and in services and large differences among geographic regions. Within any one commune, differences in family income are usually not great—at least until recently—but from county to county or from province to province major inequities, based on local conditions, persist. The "per-capita national income" in Shanghai (including its ten suburban counties whose population includes 40 percent of the municipality's total of 11 million) was, for example, $1,600 in 1980, while in some northwestern provinces and autonomous regions, it was only about $100.[23]

Furthermore, although Deng Xiaoping announced in August 1980 the goal of raising China's per capita GNP to $1,000 by the end of the century, there is no indication that the current goal includes concomitant diminution of national inequalities in wealth and income. Quite the contrary, according to China's leading economic planner, Xue Muqiao: ". . . differences in prosperity are so great, sometimes in terms of centuries, that it is impossible for all provinces and counties to join the front ranks of the world at once. The problem is that by the end of the century, 70 to 80 percent of the population will still remain poor."[24]

What would it mean for China and its people for some areas to "join the front ranks of the world" while most "still remain poor"? Current Chinese doctrine is to accept differentials in income and in growth of income on the grounds that the "to each according to his work" principle will encourage increased national productivity and therefore bring better living standards for everyone. But there are clearly problems in this approach. The idea that the benefits of increasing productivity will trickle down from a leading elite to the poor people of the society has failed in most developing countries, whose differentials of wealth remain as great or greater than before development began.

As we write this final chapter in October 1981 it is precisely 32 years since the founding of the People's Republic of China, since that portentous day when Mao Zedong stood in Tiananmen Square and proclaimed that the Chinese people had "stood up." It is a striking coincidence that October 1949 was precisely 32 years after the October Revolution, the taking of power by the Bolsheviks in Petrograd. Over the now 64 years of its history, the leadership of the Soviet Union has clearly brought about a more egalitarian redistribution of wealth and income within its society, provided access to previously unavailable health care, child care, and educational services, and built an industrial state; but, along with these achievements, a severe price has been paid. Development in the rural areas has been largely sacrificed to permit urban industrial development. A new elite takes important perquisites, perpetuates itself, and provides for its children in ways that—while certainly less inequitable than the old feudal and capitalist elites—remains clearly inequitable. There is repression of public criticism and of those wishing to emigrate, including the apparent use of the mental health system as an instrument of social and political control. An almost completely socialized health care system is unable to prevent a paradoxically rising (or at least not declining) infant mortality rate and a death rate among middle-aged men three times that of women the same age.[25]

Other countries whose governments call themselves "socialist" have developed very different models. The vast differences among Cuba, Hungary, Mozambique, and Yugoslavia, to select just a few examples, and the changes in Poland, France, and Greece as we write these words suggest that there will be a wide variety of forms of further socialist development. As China enters its next 32 years, the question of return to feudal or capitalist forms—a part of China's so recent past—is apparently settled. China's future will, so far as anyone can now tell, be a socialist one. The issue is the form that socialism will take. As the Chinese economist Xue Muqiao has recently written in *China's Socialist Economy,* a book that is one of China's best sellers, with over 2 million copies sold in 1980: "In a capitalist country, the mission of the working class is to destroy the old world. In a socialist country its task is to build a new world."[26] The new world that the Chinese will build will surely be quite different from the ones other "socialist" societies have built.

This new world will be fashioned in large part by decisions being made in China today. Some of the principles that led to China's unprecedented success in improving the health, nutrition, literacy, living conditions, and other aspects of the lives of its people are not in dispute: in the near future there is unlikely, for example, to be any significant private medicine, private education, or any substantial change in the policies that call for strict control on population growth and on rural-urban migration. But other decisions must be made—decisions on priorities for rural versus urban development, on public versus private initiatives and rewards, on letting some elements rise rapidly while others remain behind versus more egalitarian development, on increased provision of social services or production of consumer goods versus development of heavy industry, on use of resources for prevention of industrial pollution and promotion of workers' safety versus use of these resources to industrialize more rapidly, on health care versus medical care, and on permitting everyone the opportunity to play a role in health and human services versus their increased professionalization. There is danger, as we see it, that the perceptions of China's current leaders that they must use aspects of Western modernization models to industrialize rapidly in order to ease the lives of China's people and to protect themselves against foreign enemies will lead to sacrifice of some of the principles that have been China's unique strength and ironically may not even be effective in helping the vast majority of Chinese people to a better life.

There is evidence of continuing discussion within China about these fundamental decisions. For example, there appear to be differences of opinion about the wisdom of the key school system and the current emphasis on grades and examinations; several educators have called for a return to a system in which resources are shared more equitably among all institutions. In medicine there are reports that the plans to build a new high-technology medical complex in Peking have been indefinitely postponed. In other areas of health and human services there is evidence of discussion whether recent changes will indeed lead toward continued progress in China's providing for the health and well-being of all of its people. Perhaps of even greater importance, China's commitment to adequate nutrition and housing, basic literacy, and sanitation and safe water supply for all its people appears unabated.

In summary, we see in those areas that we have been privileged to observe over the decade—China's health and human services—evidence that many of the principles that have brought China so far so fast and that have inspired so many in the rest of the world are not lost, that they remain an important part of China's current practice even as the rhetoric and some of the policies move for the moment in other directions. We believe China may still lead the way to a pattern of development that will permit the introduction of appropriate technology and the attainment of high productivity—with a better standard of living for its one billion people—while preserving China's past strengths and revolutionary principles. For the sake of the Chinese people, and of the other four fifths of humankind who share a small planet with them and who may be able to learn from their accomplishments, we wish them well.

Appendices
Notes
Bibliography
Index

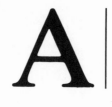

	Number	Per 10,000 Population	Number
Traditional Chinese Medical Personnel	(346,000)	(3.61)	(358,800)
Chinese Doctors (zhongyi)	251,100	2.62	257,000
Chinese Herb Specialists (zhongyao renyuan)	94,900	0.99	101,800
"Higher Level" Medical Personnel	(390,600)	(4.08)	(435,800)
Western Doctors (xiyi shi)	358,500	3.74	395,000
Pharmacologists (yaoshi)	16,700	0.17	20,000
Laboratory Doctors (jianyan shi)	7,000	0.07	9,900
Others (qita jishi)	8,400	0.09	10,900
"Middle Level" Medical Personnel	(1,064,600)	(11.11)	(1,107,700)
Assistant Doctors (yishi)	423,400	4.42	435,000
Nurses (hushi)	406,600	4.24	421,000
Midwives (zhuchan shi)	70,600	0.74	70,700
Pharmacists (yaoji shi)	67,600	0.71	76,700
Laboratory Technicians (jianyan shi)	51,500	0.54	56,200
Others (qita jishi)	44,900	0.47	48,100
"Lower Level" Medical Personnel	(662,600)	(6.92)	(737,200)
Nursing Workers (huli yuan)	180,700	1.89	218,900
Pharmacy Workers (yaoji yuan)	87,300	0.91	91,700
Laboratory Workers (jianyan yuan)	40,300	0.42	40,600
Others (qita chujie weisheng jishu renyuan)	354,300	3.70	386,000
TOTAL	2,463,900	25.72	2,642,000

Source: Ministry of Public Health, Peking, 1980 and 1981.

Professional Medical Workers in China, 1978–1980

| 79 | | 1980 | | CHANGE, 1978 to 1980 | |
Per 10,000 Population	Number	Per 10,000 Population	Change in Number	Percent Change in Number	Percent Change per 10,000 Population
(3.70)	(369,200)	(3.76)	(23,200)	(6.7)	(4.2)
2.65	262,200	2.67	11,100	4.4	1.8
1.05	107,000	1.09	12,100	12.8	9.9
(4.49)	(502,000)	(5.10)	(111,400)	(29.0)	(25.0)
4.07	447,300	4.56	88,800	24.8	21.9
0.21	25,200	0.26	8,500	50.9	47.1
0.10	14,800	0.15	7,800	111.4	106.2
0.11	14,700	0.15	6,300	75.0	70.6
(11.41)	(1,174,400)	(11.95)	(109,800)	(10.3)	(7.6)
4.48	443,800	4.52	20,400	4.8	2.2
4.34	465,800	4.74	59,200	14.6	11.8
0.73	70,800	0.72	200	0.3	−2.2
0.79	83,900	0.85	16,300	24.1	21.0
0.58	60,500	0.62	9,000	17.5	14.5
0.49	49,600	0.50	4,700	10.5	7.7
(7.60)	(752,600)	(7.66)	(90,000)	(13.6)	(10.7)
2.26	231,500	2.36	50,800	28.1	24.9
0.95	92,300	0.94	5,000	5.7	3.1
0.42	39,000	0.40	−1,300	−3.2	−5.6
3.98	389,800	3.97	35,500	10.0	7.3
27.21	2,798,200	28.50	334,300	13.6	10.8

The subtotals in this table differ slightly from the overall totals in the table and the figures used in Tables 1 and 2 because of rounding.

Barefoot Doctor Vocational Evaluation Test, Peking Municipality

(PART I)

DATE: May 13, 1979 A.M.
TIME: 2 Hours

I. Answer the following questions. (14 points)

1. What are the main physiological functions of red blood cells, white blood cells, platelets? What are their normal values? (6 points)

2. Name 5 diseases associated with hematuria. (2.5 points)

3. Name 3 pathological reflexes that are often used clinically. (3 points)

4. What are the local manifestations of general inflammation? (2.5 points)

II. What are the contraindications for preventive immunizations? (5 points)

III. There is a round well. The water is 3 meters deep and the surface is 1.5 meters in diameter. How much bleaching powder should be used for disinfection? (3 points)

IV. What are the 3 main factors for an epidemic of infectious disease? Name 2 each of gastrointestinal, respiratory, and insect-mediated infectious diseases. (6 points)

V. Describe the main diagnostic points and principles of treatment for acute gastroenteritis. (7 points)

VI. Describe the clinical manifestations and the principles of treatment of childhood rickets. (7 points)

VII. What are the symptoms and signs of acute appendicitis? What other diseases should be differentiated from it? (Name 5 diseases.) (7 points)

VIII. How many kinds of early abortion (miscarriage) are there? What are the causes of postpartum bleeding and what are the management principles? (7 points)

(PART II)

DATE: May 13, 1979 P.M.
TIME: 2 Hours

IX. How are cold diseases and hot diseases [terms from Chinese traditional medicine] diagnosed? Describe the therapeutic methods for each. (7 points)

X. What pharmaceutical categories do penicillin, streptomycin, Luminal, aspirin, sulfathiazine, piperazine, and Coramine [nikethamide] fall into? What dosage is usually used for each? Describe the precautions necessary for the use of sulfa drugs. (7 points)

Of the next six questions, select two. (15 points each)

1. What are the clinical manifestations of lobar pneumonia (including symptoms and signs, laboratory, and x-ray findings) and the therapeutic principles?

2. Describe the clinical manifestations of right heart failure. What are the therapeutic principles in the treatment of congestive heart failure? How do you use digoxin?

3. Describe the physiological functions of the organs as used in traditional Chinese medicine ["solid organs," "hollow organs"].

4. Describe the characteristics of the following pulse patterns: superficial, deep, slow, rigid, tense, slippery. What kinds of diseases do they represent?

5. Describe the characteristics of the antibacterial spectrum of penicillin. How is a skin test solution of 500 units/ml prepared from an ampule of 200,000 units? How are the results of the skin test evaluated? What is the emergency treatment for allergic shock from penicillin administration?

6. What are the 18 contradictions in the combination of traditional medicines? Give the clinical implications of the "four smells" and "five tastes" of herbal medicine.

Source: Shunyi County Hospital, June, 1980

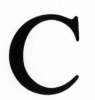

Institutes and Hospitals of the Chinese Academy of Medical Sciences and the Chinese Academy of Traditional Medicine, 1981

Chinese Academy of Medical Sciences

Peking

Institutes

Animal Center

Antibiotics

Basic Medicine—moved to Sichuan during the Cultural Revolution, now moved back to Peking

Cardiovascular Disease

Clinical Medicine

Epidemiology and Infectious Disease

Family Planning

Medical Information

Oncology (Cancer, Tumor)

Pediatrics

Pharmacology (Materia Medica)
Plastic Surgery
Public Health (Hygiene)—includes Occupational Health
Virology

Hospitals (see chapter three)

Capital—site of former Peking Union Medical College Hospital, general hospital, treats Westerners
Fuwai—cardiovascular disease
Plastic Surgery
Ritan—cancer

Medical Library
Shanghai

Parasitology Institute

Tianjin

Hematology Institute—moved to Sichuan during the Cultural Revolution, now being moved back to Tianjin

Jiangsu (Taizhou)

Dermatology Institute—will move to Nanjing

Sichuan

Biomedical Engineering Institute (formerly Medical Instrumentation)—will probably move to Tianjin
Blood Transfusion Institute (in Chengdu)
Radiation Medicine Institute—moved to Sichuan during the Cultural Revolution, will probably move back to Peking

Yunnan (Kunming)

Medical Biology Institute

Chinese Academy of Traditional Medicine

Peking

Acupuncture and Moxibustion Institute
Theoretical Basis of Traditional Medicine Institute
Traditional Pharmacology Institute

Shanghai

Traditional Medicine Institute

Source: Dr. Huang Jiasi, President, Chinese Academy of Medical Sciences, November 1981.

D | Medical Colleges in China, 1980

Provinces

Anhui	Anhui Medical College (in Hefei)
	Anhui Traditional Medical College (in Hefei)
	Bengbu Medical College
	Wannan (Anhui South) Medical College (in Wuhu)
Fujian	Fujian Medical University (in Fuzhou)
	Fujian Traditional Medical College (in Fuzhou)
Gansu	Gansu Traditional Medical College (in Lanzhou)
	Lanzhou Medical College
Guangdong	Guangdong Medical and Pharmaceutical College (in Guangzhou [Canton])
	Guangzhou Traditional Medical College
	Guangzhou Army Medical College††
	Guangzhou Medical College
	Zhanjiang Medical College
	Zhongshan (Sun Yat-sen) Medical College† (in Guangzhou)
Guizhou	Guiyang Medical College
	Guiyang Traditional Medical College
	Zunyi Medical College
Hebei	Chengde Medical Specialty School
	Hebei Medical College (in Shijiazhuang)

	Tangshan Medical College for the Coal Industry
	Zhangjiakou Medical Specialty School
Heilongjiang	Harbin Medical University
	Heilongjiang Traditional Medical College (in Harbin)
	Jianmuxin Medical College
	Jijihar Medical Specialty School
	Mudanjiang Medical Specialty School
Henan	Henan Medical College (in Zhengzhou)
	Henan Traditional Medical College (in Zhengzhou)
	Kaifeng Medical Specialty School
	Luoyang Medical Specialty School
	Yubei (Henan North) Medical Specialty School (in Ji County)
Hubei	Hubei Medical College (in Wuhan)
	Hubei Traditional Medical College (in Wuhan)
	Enzu Medical Specialty School (in Enzu County)
	Yichang Medical Specialty School
	Wuhan Medical College
	Wuhan Medical Specialty School for the Metallurgical Industry
Hunan	Hunan Medical College (in Changsha)
	Hunan Traditional Medical College (in Changsha)
	Hengyang Medical College
Jiangsu	Nanjing Medical College
	Suzhou Medical College
	Nantong Medical College
	Xuzhou Medical College
	Nanjing Railway Medical College
	Nanjing Pharmaceutical College
	Nanjing Traditional Medical College
	Yangzhou Medical Specialty School
	Zhenjiang Medical Specialty School††
Jiangxi	Jiangxi Medical College (in Nanchang)
	Jiangxi Traditional Medical College (in Nanchang)
	Gannan (Jiangxi South) Medical Specialty School (in Ganzhou)
Jilin	Bethune Medical University (in Changchun)
	Jilin Medical College (in Jilin)

	Changchun Traditional Medical College
	Yanbian Medical College (in Yanji)
Liaoning	China Medical University (in Shenyang)
	Dalian Medical College (in Dalian)
	Liaoning Traditional Medical College (in Shenyang)
	Shenyang Pharmaceutical College
	Jinzhou Medical College
	Shenyang Medical Specialty School
Qinghai	Qinghai Medical Specialty School (in Xining)
Shaanxi	Xian Medical College
	Xian Army Medical College††
	Shaanxi Traditional Medical College (in Xianyang)
	Huashan Metallurgy Medical Specialty School (in Huayi)
	Yan'an Medical College††
Shandong	Qingdao Medical College
	Shandong Medical College (in Jinan)
	Shandong Traditional Medical College (in Jinan)
	Changwei Medical College (in Weifang)
	Jining Medical Specialty School (in Jining)
	Yixue Medical Specialty School (in Yixue County)
	Heze Medical Specialty School (in Heze County)
Shanxi	Shanxi Medical College (in Taiyuan)
	Datong Medical College
	Jindongnan (Shanxi Southeast) Medical Specialty College (in Changzhi)
Sichuan	Sichuan Medical College† (in Chengdu)
	Chongqing Army Medical College††
	Chongqing Medical College
	Chengdu Traditional Medical College
	Nanchong Medical Specialty School
	Luzhou Medical College
Yunnan	Kunming Medical College
	Yunnan Traditional Medical College (in Kunming)
Zhejiang	Zhejiang Medical University (in Hangzhou)
	Zhejiang Traditional Medical College (in Hangzhou)
	Wenzhou Medical College

Autonomous Regions

Guangxi	Guangxi Medical College (in Nanning)
	Guangxi Traditional Medical College (in Nanning)
	Guilin Medical Specialty School
	Shijiang Nationalities Medical College
	(in Baise [Hundred Flowers] County)
Inner	Inner Mongolia Medical College (in Huhehot)
Mongolia	Baotou Medical College
	Zhelimu Medical College (in Tongliao)
Ningxia	Ningxia Medical College (in Yinchuan)
Tibet	Tibet Medical College (in Linzhi, near Lhasa)
Xinjiang	Xinjiang Medical College (in Urumqi)
	Shihezi Medical College

Municipalities

Peking	China Capital Medical University†
	Peking Medical College†
	Peking Second Medical College
	Peking Traditional Medical College†
	Peking Military Medical College††
Shanghai	Shanghai First Medical College†
	Shanghai Second Medical College
	Shanghai Traditional Medical College
	Shanghai Army Medical College††
	Shanghai Railway Medical College††
Tianjin	Tianjin Medical College
	Tianjin Traditional Medical College
	Tianjin Medical Specialty School

---

*Sources: The institutions in this appendix, with a few exceptions, are listed in *China Encyclopedia Yearbook,* 1980, pp. 554–558 (*yike daxue* is translated as "medical university"; *yixue yuan* as "medical college" or "medical institute"; *yixue zhuanke xuexiao* as "medical specialty school"). Those not listed in the *Yearbook* were identified in interviews in 1980 and 1981. Additional information on many of these institutions may be found in *World Directory of Medical Schools,* Fifth Edition (Geneva: World Health Organization, 1979), pp. 60-66.
† "Key" medical college.
†† Medical college not listed in *Yearbook.*

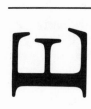 Reported Cases of Selected Infectious Diseases in China, 1978-1980

Disease	1978 Cases (in 1,000's)	1978 Deaths	1979 Cases (in 1,000's)	1979 Deaths	1980 Cases (in 1,000's)	1980 Deaths
Diseases for Which Effective Immunization Exists						
Measles	1,113	6,200	900	5,900	570	3,900
Whooping Cough (Pertussis)	595	1,000	401	700	316	400
Diphtheria	20	1,700	17	1,300	10	900
Poliomyelitis	10	260	5	140	7	170
Other Infectious Diseases						
Malaria	3,096	130	2,385	100	3,300	60
Influenza	2,659	470	2,655	360	2,938	560
"Dysentery"	2,640	6,200	2,908	6,300	2,874	4,200
Viral Hepatitis	411	1,100	472	1,100	475	1,200
Typhoid and Typhus	81	350	61	280	74	280

Source: Ministry of Public Health, Peking, 1980 and 1981.

F | Key Universities in China, 1980

Peking
Peking University
Qinghua University
China People's University
Peking Normal University
China Capital Medical University
Peking Medical College
Peking College of Traditional
    Chinese Medicine
Peking Foreign Trade Institute
Peking Foreign Languages
    Institute
Central Conservatory of Music
Central Institute of Nationalities
Northern Jiaotong University
Peking Aeronautics Institute
Peking Industrial Institute
Peking Iron and Steel Institute
Peking Institute of Posts
        and Telecommunications

Peking Institute of
    Chemical Industry
Peking Institute of
    Agricultural Machinery
Peking Agricultural University
Peking Forestry Institute
Institute of International
    Relations
Peking Sports Institute

Shanghai
Fudan University
Tongji University
Shanghai Jiaotong University
Shanghai First Medical College
Shanghai Foreign Languages
    Institute
Shanghai Normal University
Shanghai Institute of
    Chemical Industry
Shanghai Textile Institute

Tianjin
Nankai University
Tianjin University

Anhui
Chinese University of Science
and Technology
Hefei Industrial College

Fujian
Xiamen (Amoy) University

Gansu
Lanzhou University

Guangdong
Zhongshan University
Zhongshan Medical College
South China Industrial Institute
South China Agricultural
Institute

Hebei
North China Institute
of Electric Power

Heilongjiang
Harbin Industrial College
Harbin Shipping Engineering
Institute
Northeast Heavy Machinery
Institute
Daqing Petroleum Institute

Hubei
Wuhan University
Central China Industrial Institute
Wuhan Institute of
Hydroelectric Power
Wuhan Institute of Cartography
Wuhan Institute of Geology

Wuhan Building
Materials Institute
Central China Agricultural
Institute

Hunan
Xiangtan University
Hunan University
South Central Institute
of Metallurgy
Changsha Institute of
Technology

Inner Mongolia
Inner Mongolia University

Jiangsu
Nanjing University
Nanjing Industrial Institute
East China Institute
of Water Power
Nanjing Institute of Meteorology
Nanjing Aeronautics Institute
East China Engineering Institute
Nanjing Agricultural Institute
Zhenjiang Institute of
Agricultural Machinery

Jiangxi
Jiangxi Communist Labor
University

Jilin
Jilin University
Jilin Industrial College
Changchun Geology Institute

Liaoning
Dalian Industrial Institute
Northeast Industrial Institute

Dalian Ocean Shipping Institute
Shenyang Agricultural Institute
Fuxin Mining Institute

Shaanxi
Northwest University
Xian Jiaotong University
Northwest Industrial University
Northwest Telecommunications
    Engineering Institute
Northwest Light Industrial
    Institute
Northwest Agricultural Institute

Shandong
Shandong University
Shandong Oceanography
    Institute
East China Petroleum Institute

Shanxi
Shanxi Agricultural College

Sichuan
Sichuan University
Sichuan Medical College
Chongqing University
Chengdu University of Science
    and Technology
Southwest Jiaoting University
Southwest Agricultural Institute
Chinese Institute of Mining
Chengdu Telecommunications
    Engineering Institute
Chongqing Construction
    Engineering Institute

Xinjiang
Xinjiang University

Yunnan
Yunnan University

Zhejiang
Zhejiang University

Source: China Encyclopedia Yearbook, 1980.

G | Institutes of the Chinese Academy of Social Sciences, 1980

Institute of Marxism-Leninism,
    Mao Zedong Thought
Institute of Philosophy
Institute of Economics
Institute of Industrial
    Economics
Institute of Agricultural
    Economics
Institute of Finance, Trade and
    Resource Economics
Institute of World Economics
Institute of Literature
Institute of Foreign Literature
Institute of Linguistics
Institute of History
Institute of Modern History
Institute of World History
Institute of Archeology
Institute of Nationalities
Institute of Law
Institute of World Politics

Institute of World Religion
Institute of Southeast
    Asian Studies
Institute of Journalism
Institute of Information
Institute of Japanese Studies
Institute of Soviet Studies
Institute of Latin American
    Studies
Institute of African Studies
Institute of American Studies
Institute of National Minority
    Literature (Preparatory
    Group)
Institute of Sociology
    (Preparatory Group)
Institute of Political Science
    (Preparatory Group)

Source: China Encyclopedia
Yearbook, 1980.

Notes

Introduction

1. Edgar Snow, *Red China Today* (New York: Vintage, 1970).
2. Joshua S. Horn, *Away With All Pests: An English Surgeon in People's China* (New York: Monthly Review Press, 1964).
3. For example, Theodore F. Fox, "The New China: Some Medical Impressions," *The Lancet* 2 (1957): 935-39, 995-99, 1053-57; R. K. C. Thomason, W. C. MacKenzie, and A. F. W. Pert, "A Visit to the People's Republic of China," *Canadian Medical Association Journal* 97 (1967): 349-60.
4. *Gallup Poll, Public Opinion 1957-71*, Vol. III (New York: Random House, 1972), p. 2015; *Gallup Poll, Public Opinion 1972–77*, Vol. I (Wilmington, Del.: Scholarly Resources, Inc., 1978), p. 20.
5. World Bank, *World Development Report 1981* (New York: Oxford University Press, 1981).
6. Kenneth Newell, ed., *Health By the People* (Geneva: World Health Organization, 1975); V. D. Djukanovic and E. P. Mach, eds., *Alternative Approaches to Meeting Basic Health Needs in Developing Countries* (Geneva: World Health Organization, 1975); "Traditional Medicine," Special Issue of *World Health* (November 1977); Primary Health Care," Special Issue of *World Health* (April 1975);

Halfdan Mahler, "Health for All by the Year 2000," *WHO Chronicle* 29 (1975): 457-61.
7. Hossain A. Ronaghy and Steven Salter, "Is the Chinese 'Barefoot Doctor' Exportable to Rural Iran?" *The Lancet* 1(1974): 1331-3.
8. Ling Yang, "Reforming Written Chinese," *Beijing Review* 23 (August 18, 1980): 19-26.

Part I. From Mao to Modernization

Chapter 1: The Political Pendulum, 1971–1981

1. Mao Zedong, "June 26 'Directive' (June 26, 1965)," *Red Medical Battle Bulletin and August 18 Battle Bulletin Commemorative Issue* (June 26, 1967), translated in *Survey of China Mainland Press* 198 supplement (1967), p. 30.
2. Roger Garside, *Coming Alive: China after Mao* (New York: Mc-Graw-Hill, 1981), p. 48.
3. "Power Play . . . or Continuing Revolution," Interview with Paul T. K. Lin, *New China* 17 (1977): 55-62.
4. "'People's Daily' Article Repudiates Gang of Four's Absurdities on Socialist Principle 'To Each According to His Work,'" *Xinhua (New China News Agency) Weekly Issue 482* (May 11, 1978).
5. Parris H. Chang, "Chinese Politics: Deng's Turbulent Quest," *Problems of Communism* (January-February 1981): 1-21.
6. James P. Sterba, "Newspaper in Peking Lowers Mao's Pedestal a Bit," *The New York Times,* March 20, 1981.
7. Henry Kamm, "Peking Says Mao's Merits Outweigh His Mistakes," *The New York Times,* April 12, 1981.
8. James P. Sterba, "A Judgment on Mao Said To Be Reached," *The New York Times,* May 1, 1981.
9. Chang, "Chinese Politics."
10. James P. Sterba, "Successor of Mao Replaced in Peking as Party Chairman," *The New York Times,* June 30, 1981.
11. Roland Berger, "China's Economic Development Strategy," *Eastern Horizon* 19 (1980): 5-14.
12. Berger, "China's Economic Development Strategy."
13. James P. Sterba, "Chinese Shedding Proud Facade, Seek Foreign Aid," *The New York Times,* March 10, 1981.

Part II. Health Care Services

Chapter 2: Four Millennia of Medicine

1. Ilza Veith, translator, *The Yellow Emperor's Classic of Internal Medicine*, New Edition (Berkeley: University of California Press, 1972).

2. Joseph Needham, "China and the Origins of Immunology," *Eastern Horizon* 19 (1980): 6-12.

3. Needham, "China and the Origins of Immunology."

4. T'ao Lee, "Medical Ethics in Ancient China," *Bulletin of the History of Medicine* 13 (1943): 268-77.

5. Ralph C. Croizier, *Traditional Medicine in Modern China* (Cambridge, Mass.: Harvard University Press, 1968), pp. 14-15, 208.

6. John Z. Bowers, *Western Medicine in a Chinese Palace: Peking Union Medical College, 1917–1951* (New York: Josiah Macy, Jr., Foundation, 1972), p. 25; E. Richard Brown, "Exporting Medical Education: Professionalism, Modernization, and Imperialism," *Social Science and Medicine* 13A (1979):585-95; Mary Brown Bullock, *An American Transplant: The Rockefeller Foundation and Peking Union Medical College* (Berkeley, Calif.: University of California Press, 1980).

7. Bowers, *Western Medicine in a Chinese Palace*, p. 33.

8. Bertrand Russell, *The Problem of China* (New York: Norton, 1946), p. 221.

9. John B. Grant, "Rural Reconstruction in China," in *Health Care for the Community: Selected Papers of Dr. John B. Grant*, ed. Conrad Seipp (Baltimore: The Johns Hopkins Press, 1963): pp. 148-54.

10. Victor W. Sidel and Ruth Sidel, *Serve the People: Observations on Medicine in the People's Republic of China* (Boston: Beacon Press, 1974).

11. People's Republic of China, State Statistical Bureau, *Ten Great Years* (Peking: Foreign Languages Press, 1960), p. 222.

12. Additional material on the *feldsher* may be found in Victor W. Sidel, "Feldshers and 'Feldsherism': The Role and Training of the Feldsher in the Soviet Union," *New England Journal of Medicine* 278 (April 25 and May 2, 1968): 934-39, 987-92; Patrick B.

Storey, *The Soviet Feldsher as a Physician's Assistant,* DHEW Publication No. 72-58 (Washington: U.S. Government Printing Office, 1972); *The Training and Utilization of Feldshers in the USSR,* Public Health Paper No. 56 (Geneva: World Health Organization, 1974).

13. *Ten Great Years,* p. 222.

14. Leo Orleans, "Medical Education and Manpower in Communist China, *Aspects of Chinese Education,* ed. C. T. Hu (New York: Teachers College Press, Columbia University, 1969), p. 21; Chu-yuan Cheng, "Health Manpower: Growth and Distribution," *Public Health in the People's Republic of China,* eds. Myron E. Wegman, Tsung-yi Lin, and Elizabeth F. Purcell (New York: Josiah Macy, Jr. Foundation, 1973): 139-57.

15. People's Republic of China, State Statistical Bureau, "Communiqué on Fulfillment of China's 1980 National Economic Plan," *Beijing Review* 24 (May 18, 1981) : 17-20.

16. *Ten Great Years,* p. 220.

17. Chen Wen-chieh and Ha Hsien-wen, "Medical and Health Work in New China," unpublished talk given by two Chinese physicians during a visit to Canada, November 1971.

18. *China Encyclopedia Yearbook, 1980* (Peking: China Encyclopedia Publishing House, 1980), p. 559.

19. State Statistical Bureau, "Communiqué on Fulfillment of China's 1980 National Economic Plan."

20. Horn, *Away With All Pests,* p. 96.

21. Croizier, *Traditional Medicine in Modern China,* pp. 153-88.

22. David M. Lampton, *The Politics of Medicine in China: The Policy Process, 1949–1977* (Boulder, Col.: Westview Press, 1977), pp. 45-47.

23. Lampton, *Politics of Medicine,* p. 83.

24. Cheng, "Health Manpower: Growth and Distribution," p. 153.

Chapter 3: Shoes for the Barefoot Doctor?

1. *China Encyclopedia Yearbook, 1980,* p. 626.

2. A detailed description of the selection, training, and role of barefoot doctors is given in Victor W. Sidel, "The Barefoot Doctors of

the People's Republic of China," *New England Journal of Medicine* 286 (1972): 1292-99.

3. "The Orientation of the Revolution in Medical Education as Seen in the Growth of 'Barefoot Doctors,'" *China's Medicine* (October 1968): 574-81.

4. Teh-wei Hu, "Health Care Services in China's Economic Development," *China's Development Experience in Comparative Perspective,* ed. Robert F. Dernberger (Cambridge, Mass.: Harvard University Press, 1980), pp. 229-57; Teh-wei Hu, "The Financing and the Economic Efficiency of Rural Health Services in the People's Republic of China," *International Journal of Health Services* 6 (1976): 239-49.

5. Garside, *Coming Alive: China after Mao,* p. 71.

6. "Facts and Figures on China's Medical Work," *China Reconstructs* 30 (April 1981): 69-70.

7. "Ten Thousand Beijing Barefoot Doctors Take Exams," *Xinhua News Agency* (August 26, 1979).

8. Hu, "Health Care Services in China's Economic Development."

9. Hu, "Health Care Services in China's Economic Development."

10. Changwei Administrative Region Revolutionary Committee, Shandong Province, "Thriving Cooperative Medical Service," *Chinese Medical Journal* (Chinese Edition), No. 6 (June 1974): 88-89.

11. Lin Yang, "Medical and Health Services," *Beijing Review* 23 (June 23, 1980): 17-27.

12. Coordinating Study Group on the Physical Development of Children and Adolescents and Institute of Pediatrics of the Chinese Academy of Medical Sciences, "Studies on Physical Development of Children and Adolescents in New China," *Chinese Medical Journal* 3 (November 1977): 364-72.

13. "The Constitution of the People's Republic of China (Adopted March 5, 1978)," *Peking Review* 21 (March 17, 1978): 5-14.

14. Hsueh Chin-ping, Sung Hsin-ying, Ku Hsiao-chih, and Ching Ko-hsien, "An Experimental Study on the Organization of Urban Child Health Services," *Chinese Medical Journal* 84 (September 1965): 563-70.

15. Coordinating Study Group, "Studies on Physical Development

of Children and Adolescents in New China."

16. *Child Health Care in New China* (Peking: Chinese Medical Association, 1973). Reprinted in *American Journal of Chinese Medicine* 2 (1974): 149-58.

17. Hu, "Health Care Services in China's Economic Development."

18. Lael Wertenbaker, "Health Care for the Billion," *Boston Globe Magazine,* May 3, 1981.

19. E. Grey Dimond, "China Opens New Medical School," letter to the editor, *New England Journal of Medicine* 302 (February 7, 1980): 355.

20. "China Creates Acupunctural Anesthesia," *Peking Review* 14 (August 13, 1971): 7-9; *Acupuncture Anesthesia* (Peking: Foreign Languages Press, 1972).

21. Louis Lasagna, "Herbal Pharmacology and Medical Therapy in the People's Republic of China," *Annals of Internal Medicine* 83 (December 6, 1975): 887-93.

22. Chow Ying-ch'ing et al., "The Integration of Modern and Traditional Chinese Medicine in the Treatment of Fractures: IV. Treatment of Colles' Fractures," *Chinese Medical Journal* 83 (July 1964): 425-29.

23. "China Produces 3,000 Types of Traditional Chinese Medicine," *Chinese Medical Journal* 93 (December 1980): 826; Chang Hsiang-tung, "Acupuncture Analgesia Today," *Chinese Medical Journal* 92 (January 1979): 7-16.

24. Cardiovascular Section, Acupuncture Research Institute, Academy of Traditional Chinese Medicine, "Acupuncture in Coronary Heart Disease: A Report of 44 Cases," *Chinese Medical Journal* 94 (February 1981): 81-84.

25. Lin Yang, "Traditional Medicine in China Today," *Beijing Review* 23 (December 15, 1980): 21-25; "New Drug for Malaria," *Beijing Review* 21 (September 29, 1978): 27; "Yunnan Institute Develops Anti-clotting Drug," *Xinhua Weekly Issue* 651 (August 6, 1981): 14; "Breathing Exercises Help Some Blood Pressure Patients," *Xinhua Weekly Issue* 652 (August 13, 1981): 6; "Chinese-Medicine Diagnostic Computer," *Beijing Review* 24 (September 28, 1981): 29.

26. Revolutionary Committee of the Shanghai First Medical College,

"Medical Education Must be Transformed on the Basis of Mao Tse-tung's Thought," *China's Medicine* (March 1968): 159-63.

27. "China's Khrushchev Resurrected PUMC to Advance Revisionist Line in Education," *China's Medicine* (December 1967): 890-902.

28. John F. Bowers, "Medicine in Mainland China: Red and Rural," *Current Scene: Developments in Mainland China* 8 (June 15, 1970): 1.

29. Revolutionary Committee of the "June 26th" Commune of the Shantung Medical College, "A New Approach to Medical Education," *China's Medicine* (May 1968): 292.

30. Tsung O. Cheng, "Medical Education in Modern China: An Update," *Annals of Internal Medicine* 92 (May 1980): 702-04.

31. Dimond, "China Opens New Medical School."

32. "Facts and Figures on China's Medical Work," *China Reconstructs.*

33. "Importance of Nursing Work," *Beijing Review* 24 (July 13, 1981): 8, 28.

Chapter 4: Put Prevention First!

1. Leo A. Orleans and R. P. Suttmeier, "The Mao Ethic and Environmental Quality," *Science* 170 (1970): 1173-76.

2. "Environmental Protection," *Beijing Review* 23 (March 24, 1980): 5-6.

3. "Environmental Protection," *Beijing Review* 23 (September 22, 1980): 7.

4. "China's First Environmental Protection Law," *Beijing Review* 22 (November 9, 1979): 24.

5. "China's Heavy Industrial Province Makes Anti-Pollution Achievements," *Xinhua Weekly Issue* 598 (July 31, 1980): 6.

6. "Dalian Factories Fined for Pollution," *Xinhua Weekly Issue* 600 (August 14, 1980): 11.

7. Hsuchow Health and Anti-Epidemic Station, Hsuchow Coal Mining Administration, Chuantai Coal Mine and Hsuchow Medical College, "New Air-Water Jet Dust Suppressor for Coal Mines," *Chinese Medical Journal* 4 (January 1978): 47-50.

8. Liu Lisheng, Ling Yan, Tao Shouqi, and Wang Jinguan, "A Five-

Year Follow-Up Study of Hypertension in 10,450 Steel Workers," *Chinese Medical Journal* 92 (October 1979): 719-22.

9. Herbert K. Abrams, "Occupational Medicine in the People's Republic of China," *Journal of Occupational Medicine* 22 (August 1980): 553-57.

10. "Sanatoriums for Chinese Workers," *Chinese Medical Journal* 93 (December 1980): 826.

11. "Curb on Smoking," *Beijing Review* 33 (August 17, 1979): 7-8.

12. Fox Butterfield, "China Plans Campaign to Warn Against Smoking," *The New York Times,* August 5, 1979.

13. Carl Djerassi, "Steroid Contraceptives in the People's Republic of China," *New England Journal of Medicine* 289 (1973): 533-35.

14. Gerald Chen, "Population Forecasts for China's Coming Century," *Eastern Horizon* 19 (April 1980): 29-31.

15. Carl Djerassi, "The Politics of Contraception: The View from Beijing," *New England Journal of Medicine* 303 (August 7, 1980): 334-36.

16. "Report on a Talk to Rural Cadres and Commune Members on Family Planning," *Xinhua Beijing Domestic Service* (May 16, 1980). Translated in *Foreign Broadcast Information Service Daily Reports: People's Republic of China* (May 22, 1980): L7; "Population Growth Rate Declines," *Eastern Horizon* 20 (March 1981): 8; "Population Growth Declines in Chinese Provinces," *Xinhua Weekly Issue* 642 (June 4, 1981): 8.

17. Betsy Nicholas, "Birth Control in China," *Albert Einstein College of Medicine Community Health Newsletter* (December 1979): 10.

18. Shijiazhuang Hebei Provincial Service (June 30, 1980). Translated in *Foreign Broadcast Information Service Daily Reports: People's Republic of China* (July 11, 1980).

19. Djerassi, "The Politics of Contraception: The View from Beijing."

20. Nicholas, "Birth Control in China."

21. "China 'Revaluating' Daughters," *Intercom,* June/July 1979.

22. "Medical Experts Advocate Eugenics, Birth Control," *Xinhua Beijing Domestic Service* (August 22, 1980). Translated in *Foreign Broadcast Information Service Daily Reports: People's Republic of China* (August 27, 1980): L14-15.

23. "Genetic Counselling Outpatient Service," *Beijing Review* 23 (February 18, 1980): 28.

24. "Medical Experts Advocate Eugenics, Birth Control."
25. "China's Achievements in Birth Control," *Xinhua Weekly Issue* 421 (March 3, 1977).
26. "Population Growth Rate Drops," *Beijing Review* 24 (March 23, 1981): 8.
27. "Optimum Population," *Beijing Review* 24 (April 13, 1981): 29.
28. "Beijing Residents Enjoy a Longer Life," *Xinhua Weekly Issue* 555 (October 4, 1979); "Chinese Babies Healthier," *Xinhua Weekly Issue* 642 (June 4, 1981): 8.
29. "Average Life Expectancy Doubled," *Beijing Review* 24 (March 9, 1981): 7.
30. "From 36 to 68," *Beijing Review* 24 (July 6, 1981): 4-5.
31. "Average Life Expectancy Doubled."
32. "Beijing Residents Enjoy a Longer Life."
33. Lin, "Medical and Health Services."
34. "Beijing Residents Enjoy a Longer Life."
35. Huang Guojun et al., "Diagnosis and Surgical Treatment of Early Esophageal Carcinoma," *Chinese Medical Journal* 94 (April 1981): 229-32.
36. Wu Yingkai et al., "A Five Year Report on Community Control of Hypertension, Stroke, and Coronary Heart Disease in the Shijing-shan People's Commune, Beijing," *Chinese Medical Journal* 94 (April 1981): 233-36.
37. "From 36 to 68."
38. Joe D. Wray, "Child Care in the People's Republic of China, 1973," *Pediatrics* 55 (April 1975): 539-48; 55 (May 1975): 723-34; Co-ordinating Study Group, "Studies on Physical Development."
39. "Chinese Children Taller and Heavier," *Xinhua Weekly Issue* 590 (June 5, 1980): 5.

Part III. Human Services

Chapter 5: The Individual, the Group, the Community

1. Franz Schurmann, *Ideology and Organization in Communist China* (Berkeley, California: University of California Press, 1966), p. 378.
2. Theodore Shabad, *China's Changing Map* (New York: Praeger, 1972), p. 35.

3. Schurmann, *Ideology and Organization in Communist China,* p. 399.

4. Pi-chao Chen, "Overurbanization, Rustification of Urban-Educated Youths, and Politics of Rural Transformation," *Comparative Politics* (April 1972): 361-86.

5. Gordon A. Bennett and Ronald N. Montaperto, *Red Guard: The Political Biography of Dai Hsiao-ai* (Garden City, N.Y.: Anchor Books, 1972), p. 5.

6. Janet Weitzner Salaff, "Urban Residential Communities in the Wake of the Cultural Revolution," in *The City in Communist China,* ed. John Wilson Lewis (Stanford: Stanford University Press, 1971), p. 300.

7. B. Michael Frolic, *Mao's People: Sixteen Portraits of Life in Revolutionary China* (Cambridge: Harvard University Press, 1980), pp. 226-27.

8. Luo Fu, "City Dwellers and the Neighborhood Committee," *Beijing Review* 23 (November 3, 1980): 19-25.

9. Suzanne Pepper, "Chinese Education After Mao: Two Steps Forward, Two Steps Back and Begin Again?," *China Quarterly,* No. 81 (March 1980): 1-65.

10. "Job Training for Youth in China," *Eastern Horizon* 19 (October 1980): 20.

11. "Study and Job Opportunities for Youth," *Beijing Review* 23 (October 20, 1980): 28.

12. Pi-chao Chen, Commentary on Article by Chen Muhua, "Birth Planning in China," *Family Planning Perspectives* 11 (November/December 1979): 348-54.

13. Luo Fu, "City Dwellers and the Neighborhood Committee."

14. "New Elections of Beijing Neighborhood Committee," *Xinhua Weekly Issue 592* (June 19, 1980).

15. Yi-Chuang Lu, "The Collective Approach to Psychiatric Practice in the People's Republic of China," *Social Problems* 26 (1978): 2-14.

16. Ilza Veith, "Psychiatric Thought in Chinese Medicine," *Journal of the History of Medicine and Allied Sciences* 10 (1955): 261-68.

17. Ilza Veith, "The Supernatural in Far Eastern Concepts of Mental Disease," *Bulletin of the History of Medicine* 37 (1963): 139-55.

18. Veith, "Psychiatric Thought in Chinese Medicine."

19. J. Cerny, "Chinese Psychiatry," *International Journal of Psychiatry* 1 (1965): 229-38.

20. Cerny, "Chinese Psychiatry."

21. Michel Oxenberg, "China: The Convulsive Society," *Headline Series* No. 203 (New York: Foreign Policy Association, 1970).

22. Xia Zhenyi and Zhang Mingyuan, "History and Present Status of Modern Psychiatry in China," *Chinese Medical Journal* 94 (1981): 227-82.

23. Arthur Kleinman and David Mechanic, "Some Observations of Mental Illness and its Treatment in the People's Republic of China," *The Journal of Nervous and Mental Disease* 167 (1979): 267-74.

24. "Beijing Psychiatrist Discusses Treatment of Mental Disorders," *Xinhua Beijing in English* (July 7, 1980). Translated in *Foreign Broadcast Information Service Daily Report: People's Republic of China* (July 9, 1980): R 1-2.

25. Kleinman and Mechanic, "Some Observations of Mental Illness and its Treatment in the People's Republic of China."

26. Xia and Zhang, "History and Present Status of Modern Psychiatry."

27. "China's Marriage Law," *Beijing Review* 24 (March 16, 1981): 24-27.

28. Pi-chao Chen, Commentary on Article by Chen Muhua.

29. Eduard B. Vermeer, "Social Welfare Provisions and the Limits of Inequality in Contemporary China," *Asian Survey* 19 (September 1979): 856-80; "Growing Old in China," *Beijing Review* 24 (October 26, 1981): 22-28.

30. "Social Welfare Institutions," *Beijing Review* 22 (November 9, 1979): 28.

31. Wu Houde and Tian Sansong, "Well-Being of the Deaf-Blind in China," *Beijing Review* 24 (January 26, 1981): 21-25.

32. Melanie Kirkpatrick, "Blind Woman's Story, A Profile in Courage," *The Asian Wall Street Journal Weekly,* May 18, 1981.

33. Wu Houde and Tian Sansong, "Well-Being of the Deaf-Blind in China."

34. Ximen Lusha, "New Hope for Handicapped Children," *China Reconstructs* 29 (November 1980): 50-52, 70.

Chapter 6: The Family and Child Care

1. William Hinton, *Fanshen* (New York: Vintage Books, 1966).
2. Ichisada Miyazaki, *China's Examination Hell: The Civil Service Examinations of Imperial China* (New Haven: Yale University Press, 1981), p. 11.
3. Jack Belden, *China Shakes the World* (New York: Monthly Review Press, 1949), pp. 275-307.
4. "China's Marriage Law," *Beijing Review.*
5. Tan Manni, "Why the New Marriage Law Was Necessary," *China Reconstructs* 30 (March 1981): 17-23.
6. Judith Stacey, "Toward a Theory of Family and Revolution: Reflections on the Chinese Case," *Social Problems* 26 (June 1979): 499-508.
7. Martin K. Whyte, *Small Groups and Political Rituals in China* (Berkeley: University of California Press, 1975), p. 96.
8. C. K. Yang, *A Chinese Village in Early Communist Transition* (1959) in *Chinese Communist Society: The Family and the Village* (Cambridge, Mass.: M.I.T. Press, 1969), p. 117.
9. Yang, *A Chinese Village in Early Communist Transition*, p. 118.
10. Mark Selden, *The Yenan Way in Revolutionary China* (Cambridge, Mass.: Harvard University Press, 1971), p. 10.
11. A. S. Makarenko, *A Book for Parents* (Moscow: Foreign Languages Publishing House, 1954), pp. 407-8.
12. Makarenko, p. 53.
13. Yang, *A Chinese Village in Early Communist Transition*, p. 90.
14. William Kessen, ed., *Childhood in China* (New Haven: Yale University Press, 1975), p. 5.
15. R. F. Price, *Education in Modern China* (London: Routledge & Kegan Paul, 1979), pp. 21-22.
16. *China Economic Yearbook, 1981*, Section 4, p. 206.
17. "Care for 380 Million Children," *Beijing Review* 24 (April 6, 1981): 5.
18. *China Encyclopedia Yearbook, 1980*, pp. 535-36.
19. "Leader of Women's Federation Calls for More Nurseries, Kindergartens," *Xinhua Weekly Issue* 637 (April 30, 1981): 8.

20. "Nurseries Free China's Working Mothers," *Xinhua Weekly Issue* 590 (June 5, 1980): 13.

21. Ruth Sidel, *Women and Child Care in China: A Firsthand Report* (Baltimore: Penguin Books, 1973), p. 71.

22. Mao Zedong, *Five Articles* (Peking: Foreign Language Press, 1968), pp. 3-4.

23. He Zuo, "China's Education: The Type of People It Brings Up," *Beijing Review* 23 (January 7, 1980): 17-27.

24. "Minister on China's Education," *Xinhua Weekly Issue* 606 (September 25, 1980): 3.

25. Liao Jianming, "Are Redness and Expertise a Pair of Opposites?," *Guangming Ribao* (June 26, 1980). Translated in *Foreign Broadcast Information Service Daily Report: People's Republic of China* (July 9, 1980): L7.

26. "Children Study Science," *Beijing Review* 22 (May 11, 1979): 8.

27. "Pre-school Education," *Beijing Review* 24 (May 25, 1981): 27.

28. He Zuo, "China's Education: The Type of People It Brings Up."

29. "Competition Creates 'Sense of Crisis,'" *Xinhua News Agency* (August 3, 1980). Translated in *Foreign Broadcast Information Service: People's Republic of China* (August 5, 1980): L8.

30. Zhong Peizhang, "Opening Up More Outlets for an Up-and-Coming Younger Generation," *Beijing Review* 23 (August 11, 1980): 21-26.

31. "Ideological and Moral Teaching for All Primary Schools," *Xinhua Weekly Issue* 631 (March 19, 1981): 11.

32. "Beijing Children Launch 'Do a Good Deed' Campaign," *Xinhua Weekly Issue* 577 (March 6, 1980): 22.

33. "Motherly Love," *Beijing Review* 23 (June 2, 1980): 27.

34. "China's Top-level Meeting Discusses Bringing Up of Children," *Xinhua Weekly Issue* 632 (March 26, 1981): 13-14.

Chapter 7: Education

1. Suzanne Pepper, "Education and Revolution: The 'Chinese Model' Revised," *Asian Survey* (September 1978): 852-74.

2. Pepper, "Chinese Education After Mao: Two Steps Forward, Two Steps Back and Begin Again?"

3. *China Encyclopedia Yearbook, 1980,* p. 541.

4. *China Encyclopedia Yearbook, 1980*, pp. 541-42.
5. Pepper, "Chinese Education After Mao: Two Steps Forward, Two Steps Back and Begin Again?"
6. *China Encyclopedia Yearbook, 1980*, p. 536.
7. Data in this section are taken from the *China Encyclopedia Yearbook, 1980*, pp. 536, 554-58.
8. Dale Bratton, "University Admissions Policies in China, 1970-1978," *Asian Survey* (November 1979): 1008-22.
9. Pepper, "Chinese Education After Mao: Two Steps Forward, Two Steps Back and Begin Again?"
10. Personal communication with officials at Fudan University.
11. *China Encyclopedia Yearbook, 1980*, p. 539.
12. James P. Sterba, "China's Schools to Begin Giving Advanced Degrees," *The New York Times*, June 21, 1981.
13. *China Encyclopedia Yearbook, 1980*, p. 540.
14. Robert McCormick, "Central Broadcasting and Television University," *China Quarterly*, No. 81 (March 1980): 129-36.

Part IV. China and the World's Future

Chapter 8: Which Model for Modernization?

1. Barbara J. Culliton, "Science in China," *Science* 200 (October 26, 1979): 426-30.
2. James Peck, "Revolution Versus Modernization and Revisionism: A Two-Front Struggle," in *China's Uninterrupted Revolution: From 1840 to the Present*, Victor Nee and James Peck, eds. (New York: Pantheon, 1975), p. 65.
3. Peck, "Revolution Versus Modernization and Revisionism," p. 77.
4. Paul M. Sweezy, "Theory and Practice in the Mao Period," *Monthly Review* 28 (1977): 9.
5. Fred L. Pincus, "Higher Education and Socialist Transformation in the People's Republic of China since 1970: A Critical Analysis," *Review of Radical Political Economics* 11 (Spring 1979); 24-37.
6. "Health Minister on 1981 Tasks," *Chinese Medical Journal* 94 (April 1981): 240.
7. Robert J. Blendon, "Public Health Versus Personal Medical Care:

The Dilemma of Post-Mao China," *New England Journal of Medicine* 304 (April 16, 1981): 981-83.

8. James P. Sterba, "Chinese Shedding Proud Facade."

9. James P. Sterba, "China Believed to Have Understated Scale of Drought and Flood Disasters," *The New York Times,* April 25, 1981.

10. "Why China Imports Technology and Equipment," *Peking Review* 21 (October 13, 1978): 11-13.

11. Victor W. Sidel, "Public Health in International Perspective: From 'Helping the Victim' to 'Blaming the Victim' to 'Organizing the Victim,'" *Canadian Journal of Public Health* 70 (July/August 1979): 234-39.

12. See, for example, Thomas McKeown, *The Role of Medicine: Dream, Mirage, or Nemesis?* (London; Nuffield Provincial Hospital Trust, 1976), and Ivan Illich, *Medical Nemesis: The Expropriation of Health* (New York: Pantheon, 1976). For a contrary view, see Walsh McDermott, "Medicine: The Public Good and One's Own," *Perspectives in Biology and Medicine* 21 (Winter, 1978): 167-87.

13. Victor W. Sidel and Ruth Sidel, *A Healthy State: An International Perspective on the Crisis in U.S. Medical Care* (New York: Pantheon, 1977).

14. H. Jack Geiger, "Small Futures, Sick Futures, Short Futures: Inequity and Irrelevance in U.S. Health Care Strategies," in *Working For a Healthier America,* Walter J. McNerney, ed. (Cambridge, Mass: Ballinger, 1980), pp. 157-67.

15. Victor W. Sidel, "The Need for Structural Change," in *Working For a Healthier America,* pp. 168-85.

16. E. Richard Brown, "Public Hospitals in Crisis: Their Problems and Their Options," *Health Activists' Digest* 2 (Fall 1980): 3.

17. Vicente Navarro, "The Underdevelopment of Health or the Health of Underdevelopment: An Analysis of the Distribution of Human Health Resources in Latin America," *International Journal of Health Services* 4 (1974): 5-27.

18. See, for example, Sidel and Sidel, *Serve the People,* pp. 206-07; Susan B. Rifkin, "Public Health in China: Is the Experience Relevant to Other Less Developed Nations?," *Social Science and Medicine* 7 (1973): 249-57; Johan Galtung and Fumiko Nishimura,

"Can We Learn From the Chinese People?," *World Development* 4 (1976): 883-88; Robert J. Blendon, "Can China's Health Care be Transplanted Without China's Economic Policies?" *New England Journal of Medicine* 300 (1979): 1453-8; and Susan B. Rifkin, "Health, Political Will, and Participation," *UNICEF News* 108 (1981): 3-5.

19. Ronaghy and Salter, "Is the Chinese 'Barefoot Doctor' Exportable?"

20. Oscar Gish, "The Way Forward," *World Health* (April 1975): 8-13; Oscar Gish, *Planning the Health Sector: The Tanzanian Experience* (London: Croom Helm, Ltd., 1975); W. K. Chagula and E. Tarimo, "Meeting Basic Health Needs in Tanzania," in *Health By the People,* K. W. Newell, ed. (Geneva: World Health Organization, 1975), pp. 145-68; and J. K. Nyerere, *Freedom and Socialism* (London: Oxford University Press, 1968).

21. Roberto Belmar and Victor W. Sidel, "An International Perspective on Strikes and Strike Threats by Physicians: The Case of Chile," *International Journal of Health Services* 5 (1975): 53-64; Vicente Navarro, *Medicine Under Capitalism* (New York: Prodist, 1976), pp. 33-66; and Roberto Belmar et al., "Evaluation of Chile's Health System, 1973–1976: A Communication from Health Workers in Chile," *International Journal of Health Services* 7 (1977): 531-40.

22. Newell, ed., *Health by the People;* Djukanovic and Mach, eds., *Alternative Approaches;* Kenneth W. Newell, "Health Care Development as an Agent of Change," *WHO Chronicle* 30 (1976): 181-87; Mahler, "Health for All by the Year 2000"; and Halfdan Mahler, "Bringing Down the Medical Empire," *Pan American Health* 10 (1973): 10-15.

23. "Differences Between Localities," *Beijing Review* 24 (September 14, 1981): 3.

24. "Personal Incomes in China," *The China Business Review* 8 (March-April 1981); 19-20.

25. Christopher Davis and Murray Feshbach, *Rising Infant Mortality in the U.S.S.R. in the 1970's* (Washington, D.C.: Bureau of the Census, 1980); Serge Schmemann, "Soviet Affirms Rise in Infant Mortality," *The New York Times,* June 21, 1981; Theodore Shabad, "Death Rate of Men Up in Soviet Towns," *The New York Times,* June 11, 1979.

26. Xue Muqiao, *China's Socialist Economy* (Beijing: Foreign Languages Press, 1981), p. iv; "1980 Best Sellers in China," *Eastern Horizon* 20 (March 1981): 51.

Bibliography

A Barefoot Doctor's Manual. Seattle: Cloudburst Press, 1977 (Originally published in Chinese in 1970 by the Institute of Traditional Chinese Medicine of Hunan Province).

Acupuncture Anesthesia (DHEW Publication No. (NIH) 75-784). Washington, D.C.: U.S. Government Printing Office, 1975 (Originally published in Chinese in 1972 by a group of medical institutions in Shanghai).

Andors, Stephen. *China's Industrial Revolution: Politics, Planning and Management, 1949 to the Present.* New York: Pantheon Books, 1977.

Barnett, A. Doak. *China's Economy in Global Perspective.* Washington, D.C.: The Brookings Institution, 1981.

Bowers, John F. *Western Medicine in a Chinese Palace: Peking Union Medical College, 1917–1951.* New York: Josiah Macy, Jr., Foundation, 1972.

Bowers, John F. and Purcell, Elizabeth F. *Medicine and Society in China.* New York: Josiah Macy, Jr. Foundation, 1974.

Bullock, Mary Brown. *An American Transplant: The Rockefeller Foundation and Peking Union Medical College.* Berkeley: University of California Press, 1980.

Burton, Neil G. and Bettelheim, Charles. *China Since Mao.* New York: Monthly Review Press, 1978.

Croizier, Ralph C. *Traditional Medicine in Modern China: Science, Nationalism, and the Tensions of Cultural Change.* Cambridge: Harvard University Press, 1968.

Dernberger, Robert F., ed. *China's Development Experience in Comparative Perspective.* Cambridge: Harvard University Press, 1980.

Dimond, E. Grey. *More Than Herbs and Acupuncture.* New York: Norton, 1975.

Frolic, B. Michael. *Mao's People: Sixteen Portraits of Life in Revolutionary China.* Cambridge: Harvard University Press, 1980.

Gurley, John G. *China's Economy and the Maoist Strategy.* New York: Monthly Review Press, 1976.

Herbal Pharmacology in the People's Republic of China. Washington, D.C.: National Academy of Sciences, 1975.

Horn, Joshua S. *Away With All Pests: An English Surgeon in People's China, 1954–1969.* New York: Monthly Review Press, 1969.

Hu Teh-wei, *An Economic Analysis of the Cooperative Medical Services in The People's Republic of China* (DHEW Publication No. (NIH) 75-672). Washington, D.C.: U.S. Government Printing Office, 1975.

Kao, Frederick F., and Kao, John J., eds. *Chinese Medicine–New Medicine.* Garden City, NY: Institute for Advanced Research in Asian Science and Medicine, 1977.

Kaplan, Henry S., and Tsuchitani, Patricia Joros, eds. *Cancer in China.* New York: Alan R. Liss, Inc., 1978.

Kleinman, Arthur, Kunstadter, Peter, Alexander, E. Russell; and Gale, James L. *Medicine in Chinese Cultures: Comparative Studies of Health Care in Chinese and Other Societies* (DHEW Publication No. (NIH) 75-653). Washington, D.C.: U.S. Government Printing Office, 1975.

Lampton, David M. *The Politics of Medicine in China: The Policy Process, 1949–1977.* Boulder, Col.: Westview Press, 1977.

Leslie, Charles, ed. *Asian Medical Systems: A Comparative Study.* Berkeley: University of California Press, 1976.

Nee, Victor, and Peck, James. *China's Uninterrupted Revolution: From 1840 to the Present.* New York: Pantheon, 1975.

Newell, Kenneth W., ed. *Health By The People.* Geneva: World Health Organization, 1975.

Orleans, Leo A. *Every Fifth Child: The Population of China.* Stanford: Stanford University Press, 1972.

Pepper, Suzanne. "Chinese Education After Mao: Two Steps Forward, Two Steps Back and Begin Again?" *China Quarterly,* No. 81, March 1980, pp. 1–65.

Price, Ronald F. *Education in Modern China.* London: Routledge and Kegan Paul, 1979.

Quinn, Joseph R., ed. *Medicine and Public Health in the People's Republic of China* (DHEW Publication No. (NIH) 73–67). Washington, D.C.: U.S. Government Printing Office, 1973.

Quinn, Joseph R., ed. *China Medicine As We Saw It* (DHEW Publication No. (NIH) 75–684). Washington, D.C.: U.S. Government Printing Office, 1974.

Selden, Mark. *The Yenan Way In Revolutionary China.* Cambridge: Harvard University Press, 1971.

Sidel, Victor W., and Sidel, Ruth. *A Healthy State: An International Perspective on the Crisis in U.S. Medical Care.* New York: Pantheon, 1978.

Spence, Jonathan D. *The Gate of Heavenly Peace: The Chinese and Their Revolution, 1895–1980.* New York: Viking, 1981.

United States–China Science Cooperation, Hearings Before the Subcommittee on Science, Research and Technology of the Committee on Science and Technology, U.S. House of Representatives, May 7, 8, 10, June 22, 1979. Washington, D.C.: U.S. Government Printing Office, 1979.

Wegman, Myron L.; Lin, Tsung-yi; and Purcell, Elizabeth F., eds. *Public Health in The People's Republic of China.* New York: Josiah Macy, Jr., Foundation, 1973.

World Bank. *World Development Report 1981.* New York: Oxford University Press, 1981.

Xue Muqiao. *China's Socialist Economy.* Beijing: Foreign Languages Press, 1981.

Index

Abortion, 81, 88, 229
Academy of Medical Sciences, *see*
  Chinese Academy of Medical
  Sciences
Academy of Sciences, *see* Chinese
  Academy of Sciences
Academy of Social Sciences, *see* Chi-
  nese Academy of Social Sciences
Academy of Traditional Chinese
  Medicine, *see* Chinese Academy
  of Traditional Medicine
Acupuncture, 20, 56, 59, 115, 232;
  analgesia, 60; anesthesia, 7, 59,
  60; humoral theories of action of,
  61; reports of efficacy of, 60-61;
  used for mental illness treatment,
  115, 118
Adult education, 173-174
Agriculture, modernization of, 10,
  12, 13-14, 178
All-China Federation of Trade Unions,
  77
Allende, Salvador, 199
Analgesia, acupuncture, 60
Anesthesia, acupuncture, 7, 59, 60
Anshan Iron and Steel Company,
  142-143
Assistant doctors, 29, 67, 69, 226-227

Baoshan Steelworks, 13
Barefoot doctors (*chijiao yisheng*),
  35, 46, 69, 76, 113, 184; attempt
  to introduce, into other countries,
  199; criticism of, 40; defined, 37;
  distribution of contraceptives by,
  80; examinations for, 42-44, 228-
  230; income of, 39, 44, 47; number
  of, 41-42; preservation of, 189; and
  surveys of preschool children, 98;
  tasks provided by, 38; training of,
  37-39, 40-42, 44
Beihai Kindergarten (Peking), 137
Beijing Review, 61, 108, 139, 140, 142
Bethune, Norman, 28
Birth control: campaigns, 80; methods,
  80-81, 86
Birth rate, 81
Blendon, Robert, 189
Blind people, 120-121, 122, 124
Blood pressure screening, industrial,
  76. *See also* Hypertension
Breathing: exercise, deep (*qigong*), 62;
  and gymnastic exercises, 20, 115
Bronx, New York, health services in,
  196-197
Burns, treatment for severe, 57
Butterfield, Fox, 78-79

Campaigns, health, 30-32, 72; birth
    control, 80; immunization, 31, 97;
    against opium use, 31, 115; against
    prostitution, 31, 115; against schis-
    tosomiasis, 31-32, 72; against
    smoking, 79; against venereal dis-
    ease, 31, 115
Cancer, 94-96, 98; esophagus, 95-96;
    lung, 78, 79, 95
Capital Hospital (Peking), 56, 232
Capital Iron and Steel Complex
    (Peking), 76
Capital Medical College (Peking), 57,
    67-68. *See also* China Capital
    Medical University
Central Art Institute, 158
Central Committee Plenum, Third,
    11-12
Chaoyang New Village hospital
    (Shanghai), 52-53
Chiang Kai-shek, 102
Children: impact of modernization on,
    187; improved growth and develop-
    ment of, 97-98; special attention to
    health and care of, 54-56, 184
China Blind People's Welfare Institute,
    121
China Capital Medical University
    (Peking), 58, 67-68, 236. *See also*
    Capital Medical College; China
    Medical College
China Economic Yearbook (1981), 134
China Encyclopedia Yearbook (1980),
    135
China Medical Board, 24
China Medical College (Peking), 28-
    29, 63. *See also* China Capital
    Medical University
China Medical Commission, 24
China-Rumania People's Commune
    (Peking), 41, 43
China Welfare Institute of the Deaf,
    121
China's Medicine, 63, 64, 65
Chinese Academy of Medical Sciences,
    56, 64, 68, 88, 231-232; Capital
    Medical College of, 58, 67-68; Insti-
    tute of Pediatrics of, 54-55; Labor
    Protection Section of Institute of
    Public Health of, 76-77; Oncology
    Institute of, 56

Chinese Academy of Sciences, 88,
    172-173; Graduate Academy of,
    171; Institute of Genetics of, 88
Chinese Academy of Social Sciences,
    173, 241; Graduate Academy of,
    171-172
Chinese Academy of Traditional
    Medicine, 68, 232; Acupuncture
    Research Institute of, 60-61; Insti-
    tute of Traditional Chinese Phar-
    macology of, 61
Chinese Medical Association, 63
Chinese Medical Journal, 60, 63, 75,
    76, 116-117
Ching hao su (antimalarial drug), 61
Chuantai Coal Mine, 75
Cigarettes: dangers of smoking, 78-79;
    production of, 79. *See also* Smoking
Cities, medical practice in, 49-58.
    See also Urban organization
Civic consciousness, 145
Colleges, *see* Higher education
Committee for the Defense of Children,
    85, 135, 140
Commune(s), 69, 128, 131; clinics, 33,
    44; hospitals, 44; rural, 37, 46-47,
    103; urban, 103, 104
Communists, Communist Party, 3, 9,
    12, 33, 132; Committee of, 109-
    110; and Communist Youth League,
    163; on equality of women, 127-
    128; and higher education, 166;
    policies of, on Chinese medicine,
    22; and preschool care, 147; and
    revolutionary committees, 7; ser-
    vices to cities by, 123; Third
    Plenary Session of (1978), 11-12,
    13; and urban organization, 102,
    104, 109
Communist Youth League, 79, 109,
    163
Confucianism, 131-132
Confucius, 11, 154
Contraceptives, types of, 80-81, 86
Cooperative medical services (*hezuo
    yiliao*), 46-48, 189
Costs of hospital services, 47-48; of
    medical care services, 57
Cultural and Literary Council for
    Children, 148
Cultural Revolution, 11, 14, 36, 56,

Cultural Revolution, *(cont.)*
80; and barefoot doctors, 40, 46;
central issues of, 3-4; deaths during,
5; discontinuance of work for blind
and deaf during, 121; discouraging
of aggregation of health statistics
during, 89; dissolution of trade
unions during, 77; educational
policy during, 153-154, 156, 159-
169 *passim*; emphasis on local
control and deprofessionalization
during, 52; and health care system,
27-32, 37, 46; and Hua Guofeng,
178; and human services, 7-8;
maligning of intellectuals during,
183; and medical education, 62;
mental health services during,
115-116; persecutions during,
109-110; and pollution control, 72-
73; and preschool care, 137-148
passim; productivity problems during, 184; and Red Medical Workers,
53; reforms of, 9; and rural health
care, 189; stress on antielitism and
popular participation during, 123;
and traditional medicine, 58, 60;
urban organization during, 104,
105, 108, 112; and urban and rural
health workers, 38, 39; youth sent
to countryside during, 110

Da Cheng Nursery (Peking), 138
Da Cheng Residents' Committee, 86,
111-112
Dao, Daoism, 21, 114
Daqing oil field, 9
Deaf people, 120-121, 122, 124
Death, leading causes of, 94-97. *See
also* Mortality rates
Defense, *see* Military
Deng Xiaoping, 4, 10, 13, 155, 162,
177; on barefoot doctors, 40; on
China's GNP, 204; on graduate
education, 171; and modernization,
178, 180; pragmatic ideology of,
11-12
Dewey, John, 133
Diphtheria, 55, 97, 237
District Government Arms, 108
Divorce, 129

Djerassi, Carl, 81
Doctors, *see* Assistant doctors; Barefoot doctors; Physician(s); Worker
doctors

Earthquake, Tangshan (1976), 6, 177,
191
Education: abolishment of elitism in,
8; administration of, 156-158;
graduate, 171-173; higher, 164-171;
policies, current, 14-15, 181-182,
187; policies, 1949-1976, 150-156;
primary, 158-161; secondary, 161-
163; spare-time and adult, 173-174
Education, Bureau of, 109, 142, 146
Eighth Route Army, 127
Electroshock treatment, 115, 118
Eliot, Charles, 24
Environmental and occupational
health, 72-79
Environmental Protection Office, 73
Exercise, 20, 60

Family: impact of modernization on,
185-186; one-child, 84-85, 86-87;
planning, 6, 79-89, 111, 200-201;
structure, 125-131; as three-generational unit, 128-129, 185
Feldshers, 29
Fengsheng Neighborhood (Peking),
105-106, 109-110, 112; Committee,
106-107; Hospital, 52, 54, 106,
109; population of, 109; unemployment in, 111
Food shortages, relief efforts for, 191
Foreign aid: Chinese acceptance of,
191, 192; curtailing of Chinese,
191-192
Foreign languages, teaching of, in
primary schools, 160
Four Modernizations policy, 10, 12-15,
136, 140, 159; campaign for,
178-179, 182, 183
Four Olds, attacks on, 58, 104-105
"Four pests," campaign against, 30-31
Fractures, treatment of, 20, 60
Friendship (Youyi) Hospital (Peking),
56
Fudan University (Shanghai), 169, 170

Fuzhimenwai (or Fuwai) Hospital
(Peking), 56, 232

Gang of Four, 11-12, 40, 54, 60, 110,
183; accusations against, 9-10;
arrest and overthrow of, 105, 154-
155, 166, 167, 177, 181; identified,
9; impact on health care system of,
52; and preschool education, 135;
and trade union sanatoriums and
rest homes, 77
Gao Zhizhang, 144
Ge Hong, 21
General Administrative Committee,
109, 110
Genetic counseling, 88
Genghis Khan, 11
Gongjiang Kindergarten (Shanghai),
138-139
Graduate education, 171-172; admissions to, 172; curriculum and
teaching in, 172-173
Grant, John B., 25
Great Leap Forward (1957-1958), 4,
11, 33, 37, 178; education during,
151-152, 154; goals of, 103; preschool care during, 133; termina-
tion of birth control programs
during, 80
Great Patriotic Health Campaigns,
30-31, 72, 178
Groups: neighborhood, 108; study,
113
Guozi Shi (Fruit Market) Kindergarten
(Peking), 141-142, 144

Han dynasty, 21
Handicapped people, care for, 120-
124
Hatem, George (Ma Haide), 28
Health care models: future, 203-206;
for other countries, 192-203
Health care system, 15; effect of
political upheaval of 1960s on,
4-7; prior to Liberation, 19-27;
from Liberation to Cultural Revolution, 27-32
Health policy, results of (1949-1965),
33-34

Health statistics, 89-98, 237
Health workers: education of, 62-70;
Red Cross, 53-54, 113, 189; training
of peasant, 37-39, 40-42, 44 (*see
also* Barefoot doctors); training of
professional, 29, 30; urban, in
countryside, 39, 42
Heart disease, 94, 96
Hebei Province, 1980 droughts in, 14
Hepatitis, infectious, 98, 237
Herbal medicine, 20, 59-60, 115, 118
Higher education, 164-165; adminis-
tration of, 166; admissions to, 166-
168; curriculum and teaching in,
168-170; key universities in, 165-
166; tuition and costs of, 170-171
Hinton, William, *Fanshen*, 125
Horn, Joshua, 32
Hospital(s), 56; beds, number of, 30,
45, 57; costs, 47-48; neighborhood,
51-54; psychiatric, 114-115
Hu Yaobang, 12
Hua Guofeng, 9, 10, 178; and Deng
Xiaoping, 11-12; fall from power
of, 143; on family planning, 84
Huang Hua, 11
Huangdi Neijing (*The Yellow Emperor's
Classic of Internal Medicine*), 19
Hubei Province, floods in, 14
Human services, 15; impact of modern-
ization on health and, 181, 183-
184, 188-190; provision of, 7
Hunan Medical College, 88
Hypertension, 76, 95, 96, 98

Illiteracy, 27; large-scale attack on, 30
Immunization, 55-56, 228-229; cam-
paigns, 31, 97
Income, differences in, 203-204
Industrialization, contradiction be-
tween rapid, and environment-
worker protection, 77-78
Industry, modernization of, 10, 12,
13, 178
Infant mortality rates, 26, 90-91, 97
Infectious diseases, 26, 34, 94, 97, 98,
237
Inoculation, discovery of smallpox, by
Chinese, 20-21

Institute of Labor and Occupational Health (Shanghai), 76
Insulin shock treatment, 115, 118
Insurance, medical: labor (*laobao yiliao*), 56-57; public expenses (*gongfei yiliao*), 56
International Acupuncture Training Courses, 61
International Monetary Fund, 192
International Red Cross, 14

Jenner, Edward, 20-21
Jiang Qing, 9. *See also* Gang of Four
Johns Hopkins Medical School, 26

Kindergarten, *see* Preschool care
Kuomintang (Guomindang), 102, 127

Laboratory workers/doctors/technicians, 70
Li Chaobo, 73
Li Qingshu, 122
Liberation (1949), 4, 33, 116; health care from, to Cultural Revolution, 27-32; health care prior to, 19-27
Liberation Army Daily, 11
Life expectancy, 94, 97
Lin Biao, 154
Linxian (Lin County, Henan), 95-96
Liu Shaoqi, 3, 4, 152-153, 162

Ma Hiade (George Hatem), 28
Ma Qiao (Horse Bridge) People's Commune (Shanghai), 44
MacKenzie, John Kenneth, 23
Mahler, Halfdan, 200
Malaria, 61, 97, 237
Malnutrition, 26, 94
Mao Zedong, 8, 65, 105, 115, 116, 204; his attack on Ministry of Public Health ("June 26th Directive"), 4, 38, 62; and barefoot doctors, 40; and birth control, 80; death of, 9, 105, 108, 154, 155, 177, 180; and educational policies, 134, 153, 159; evaluation of contributions of, 10-11; on foreign technology, 192; and Gang of Four, 177; and Great Leap Forward, 151; health care efforts of, 27-28, 33, 54; power struggle between Liu Shaoqi and, 3, 152-153; and preschool care, 138, 142, 144; "Serve the People," 137; tenets adopted by, 5; and uninterrupted revolution, 180, 183
Marriage, 126-127; arranged, 126, 129-130; consanguineous, 88; legal age of, 87, 129
Marriage Introduction Service, 130
Marriage Laws: (1950), 119, 128, 129; (1981), 87, 119, 129
Massachusetts General Hospital, 58
Massage, 60
Maternal and child health, 54, 87
May 4 movement (1919), 127, 150
Measles, 55, 97, 237
Medical personnel, *see* Health workers
Medical practice: in cities, 49-58; in rural areas, 36-49
Medical colleges, 28-29, 34, 233-236; analysis of (after 1966), 64-70; analysis of (prior to 1966), 62-64; closing of, 5; recruitment of workers and peasants into, 6-7; reopening of, 6
Medicine, Chinese traditional, 58-62, 229-230, 232; effect of Jesuit missionaries on, 22-23; modernization policies in, 14; principles of, 21-22; theory and techniques of, 19-21; training in, 68; used for mental illness treatments, 115, 118; and Western medicine, 7, 19, 23-24, 27, 28, 32, 58-59
Mencius, 22
Mental health services, 112-119
Mental retardation, 120, 121-123
Microsurgery, 57
Midwives, 25, 29, 69, 80, 87, 226-27
Migration, urban, 36, 103
Military (defense), modernization of, 10, 178
Ministry of Agriculture, 78-79, 165

Ministry of Education, 135, 144, 159,
    160, 162; and graduate education,
    172, 173; and higher education,
    164, 165, 168, 169; responsibilities
    of, 156, 164
Ministry of Finance, 78-79
Ministry of Foreign Affairs, 165
Ministry of (Public) Health, 4, 33-34,
    54-55, 61, 78-79, 117, 165; pub-
    lished official goals of, 188
Ministry of Higher Education, 164
Ministry of Light Industry, 78-79
Missionaries, Jesuit, 22-23
Models, see Health care models
Modernization programs, 10, 12-15,
    58; impact of, on China's society,
    177-192 passim; impact of, on
    health and human services, 181,
    183-184, 188-190. See also Four
    Modernizations policy
Montefiore Hospital (Bronx, New
    York), Community Health Partici-
    pation Program of, 201-203
Mortality rates, 26, 36, 80, 81-82, 91-
    94, 96; infant, 26, 90-91, 97
Moxibustion, 20, 60, 232

National Conference on Educated
    Youth Settling in the Countryside,
    110
National Coordinating Committee on
    Children and Youngsters' Work,
    147-148
National Council on Daily Necessities
    for Children, 148
National Health Congress, first (1950),
    28
National minorities, 68, 89
National People's Congress, 102; Fifth
    (1979), 73, 82, 83-84, 87
National Science Conference, 178
Neighborhood Agencies, 108
Neighborhood organization, 7-8;
    impact of modernization on, 186-
    187. See also Urban organization
Neighborhood or street committees,
    108
New Culture movement (1917), 127
New York Times, 56, 79, 191

Nursery schools, see Preschool care
Nurses, 29, 226-227; growth in number
    of, 45, 69; shortage of, 27
Nursing workers, 69-70, 226-227
Nutritional deficiency diseases, 97
Nyerere, Julius K., 199

Occupational health, environmental
    and, 72-79
October Revolution, 204
Oksenberg, Michel, 116
Opium use, campaigns against, 31, 115
Organization, urban, 7-8, 14, 49;
    current status of, 108-112; history
    of, 101-107; levels of, 108

Patients: differentiation of, by class,
    22; ratio of physicians to, 29, 68;
    treatment of female, 21-22
Peking Art School, 158
Peking (Beijing): barefoot doctors in,
    43, 228-230; earthquake in, 6; ed-
    ucation in, 157, 158, 170; family
    planning in, 85-86; health statistics,
    90, 94; health workers in, 45, 48-
    50; hospitals in, 56, 62, 232; hos-
    pital beds in, 48-50; hypertension
    in, 76, 96-97; institutes in, 60-61,
    77, 231-32, 241; medical care in,
    44, 54; medical colleges in, 65-67,
    76, 116, 236; mental health in,
    117; preschool care in, 135-38,
    141-42, 144-47; universities in,
    238; urban organization in, 105-12
Peking Bureau of Education, 142
Peking Bureau of Public Health, 43
Peking Foreign Languages Institute/
    School, 158
Peking Medical College, 65, 66, 67,
    116; Faculty of Public Health at,
    76
Peking Radio Domestic Service, 64
Peking Traditional Chinese Medicine
    Hospital, 62
Peking Traditional Medical College, 67
Peking Union Medical College (PUMC),
    24-25, 26, 28, 56, 58, 63-64;
    mental health services at, 114.
    See also China Medical College

Peking University, 171
Pellagra, 97
Pensions, 120
People's Daily (Renmin Ribao), 10-11, 64-65, 82
People's Liberation Army, 7, 10, 27, 105, 106, 116; and higher education, 166
Pertussis (whooping cough), 55, 97, 237
Pharmacists, pharmacologists, 29, 69, 226-227
Physician(s): appointed to courts, 21; effect of 1960s political upheaval on, 5; honor to, 22; /patient ratio, 29, 68; training of, 29
Plague, pneumonic, outbreak of, 23-24
"Planned Parenthood Glory Certificate," 84
Poliomyelitis, 55, 97, 237
Pollution: air, 73; control, 72, 73-74, 77; industrial, 73, 77, 98; water, 73, 77-78
Population: decline in (1970s), 82; estimated future growth of, 82-83, 89; growth of (1950s), 80; urban vs. rural, 36, 103
Population Reference Bureau, 91
Preschool care, 131-134; changes in, 143-145; descriptions of, 140-143; facilities for, 8, 14, 134-136; fees for, 136; goals of, 140; national activity on behalf of, 147-148; structure of, 136-139; teachers of, 145-147
Prescriptions, dispensing of secret, 22
Prevention, emphasis on, 6, 21, 71
Preventive medicine, 26, 28
Primary education, 158-161
Production brigade(s), 37, 38, 39, 41, 46, 69; health stations, 44
Production and Service Department, 109, 111
"Productive labor," 138-139, 144-145
Prostitution, campaigns against, 31, 115
Psychiatry/psychotherapy, 118-119. *See also* Mental health services
Public health, 23-24, 34; specialists, training of, 29; work in, at PUMC, 25

Public Health, Bureau of, 43, 49, 51, 109
Pulse-taking, prolonged and detailed, 20, 60
PUMC, *see* Peking Union Medical College

Qi (life force), 20
Qian Xinzhong, 188
Qigong (deep breathing exercise), 62
Qing (Ch'ing) dynasty, 22-23

Red Cross Health (Medical) Workers, 53-54, 113, 189
Red Cross Members, 53
Red Cross Societies, 53, 184, 191
Red Guards, 104-105, 138, 153, 178; Communist Youth League replaced by, 163; education of, 154
Red Medical Workers, 6, 49-51, 53, 55, 76, 189; distribution of contraceptives by, 80; in Fengsheng Neighborhood (Peking), 106
"Red" versus "expert," 8, 10, 14, 139-140, 154-155; defined, 152
Renmin Ribao, see People's Daily
Residents' committees, 102-103, 104, 106, 108; responsibilities of, 107, 109, 111-112
Respiratory disease, 96
Rest homes, trade union, 77
Reston, James, 56
Retirement, 120
Revolution, concept of uninterrupted, 180, 183
Revolutionary committees, neighborhood, 7, 105, 108
Revolutionary optimism, concept of, 115-116
Rickets, 97, 229
Ritan Hospital (Peking), 56, 232
Rites of the Zhou Dynasty, 114
Rockefeller Foundation, 24
Rural areas, medical practice in, 36-49
"Rural doctor" *(noncoun yisheng)*, 44
Rural health program, development of, 25-26
Russell, Bertrand, 25
Rustification movement, 103-104

Sanatoriums, 118; trade union, 77
Sanitarians, 29
Sanitation, 6
Schistosomiasis, campaign against,
    31-32, 72
Science and technology, modernization
    of, 10, 178
Secondary education, 161-163
"Self-reliance" (*zili gengsheng*), 5, 191
Shandong Medical College, 65
Shanghai: barefoot doctors in, 38, 43-
    44; education in, 157, 170; health
    statistics, 90, 95; health workers in,
    48-50; hospitals in, 115; hospital
    beds in, 48-50; institutes in, 76,
    121-123, 232; lung cancer in, 79;
    medical colleges in, 76, 116, 236;
    mental health in, 117; pollution in,
    72; population distribution, 83-84;
    preschool care in, 138, 140-141;
    residents' committee in, 107;
    revolutionary committees in, 105;
    universities in, 238
Shanghai Children's Welfare Institute,
    121-123
Shanghai First Medical College, 62-63,
    67; Faculty of Public Health at, 76
Shanghai Machine Tool Plant, preschool
    facility at, 140-141
Shanghai Municipal Affairs Bureau,
    121
Shanghai Municipal Revolutionary
    Committee, 72
Shanghai Normal School, 143, 144,
    146-147
Shanghai Second Welfare Institute, 123
Shanghai Shipping Bureau, 130
Shoudu, *see* Capital Hospital
Shunyi County (Peking), 41, 42, 43;
    commune hospitals and clinics in,
    44; county hospital in, 45-46
Sichuan Medical College (Chengdu), 67
Smallpox inoculation, discovery of, by
    Chinese, 20-21
Smoking, 98; absence of attempt to
    educate about dangers of, 78;
    campaign against, 79
Social mobilization, defined, 179
Social welfare services, 119-124
Society, impact of modernization on
    China's, 177-192 *passim*

Splinting, flexible, 20, 60
State Council, 73, 78, 164, 165
State Planning Commission, 79
Sterilization, male and female, 81, 86
Stomatologists, 29
Streamlining, process of, 152
Stroke, 94, 96
Subdistrict offices, 102, 104, 108
Suicides, 127
Sun Yat-sen, 11, 127
Superstition, large-scale attack on, 30
Surgery, 57
Sweezy, Paul, 182

Tangshan, 6, 177, 191
Technicians, 29, 226-27
Technology, 181; and equipment,
    foreign, 190-191, 192; moderni-
    zation of science and, 10, 178
Television University, 174
Therapeutic medicine, 26-27, 28, 32
Thyroid disease, 97
Tianjin (Tientsin): earthquake in, 6;
    health workers in, 48-50; hospital
    beds in, 48-50; institute in, 232;
    medical colleges in, 23, 236;
    universities in, 239
Tingxian (Ting County, Peking), 25
Tuberculosis, 55

Unemployment, 110-111
Unions, trade, 77, 79
United Nations, 14, 192; World Food
    Program of, 191
Universities, *see* Higher education
Urban areas, medical practice in, 49-58
Urban organization, 7-8, 14, 49;
    current status of, 108-112; history
    of, 101-107; levels of, 108

Venereal disease, 97; campaigns
    against, 31, 115

Wang Hongwen, 9. *See also* Gang of
    Four
Warring States period, 21

Women: abuse of, in pre-Liberation China, 125-127; changing role of, 127-131; impact of modernization on, 187-188; patients, treatment of, 21-22
Women's Federation, 87, 109, 136, 147, 148
Worker doctors, 75-76
World Bank, 91, 94, 192
World Health Organization, 57, 61, 96, 200
Wu, wuyi, 114
Wu Lien-teh, 23-24
Wu Min, 88
Wuting Residents' Committee (Peking), 54

Xinhua (New China) News Agency, 72, 89, 111, 145
Xue Muqiao, 204; *China's Socialist Economy*, 205
Xuzhou Coal Mining Administration, 75

Xuzhou Health and Anti-Epidemic Station, 75
Xuzhou Medical College, 75

Yang Jiezeng, 122
Yangsheng Commune (Peking), 43
Yao Wenyuan, 9, 10. *See also* Gang of Four
Yexian (Ye County, Shandong), 42
Yin and *yang*, 20, 114
Young Pioneers, 160, 163
Youyi Hospital (Peking), *see* Friendship Hospital

Zhang Chunqiao, 9. *See also* Gang of Four
Zhang Shuyi, 140
Zhongguo Funu (*Women in China*), 141
Zhongshan (Dr. Sun Yat-sen) Medical College (Guangzhou), 67, 233
Zhou Enlai, 9, 10, 69, 150, 178
Zhu De, 177

Ruth Sidel, associate professor of sociology at Hunter College, City University of New York, has traveled extensively throughout the world studying child care and human services. She is the author of numerous books and articles, including her widely acclaimed *Women and Child Care in China*.

Victor W. Sidel, M.D., is chairman of the Department of Social Medicine at Montefiore Hospital and Medical Center and professor of Community Health at the Albert Einstein College of Medicine in New York. He is a frequent consultant to the World Health Organization and has been honored by the New York Academy of Sciences for "outstanding contributions toward the improvement of the health of the population."